Sirtfood Diet

A Smart 7 Days Meal Plan to Kick-Start your "Skinny Gene", Get Lean Muscle and Burn Fat. 200 Easy and Tasty Recipes to Feel Great, Stay Fit and Enjoy the Food You Love.

Adele Middleton

Table of Contents

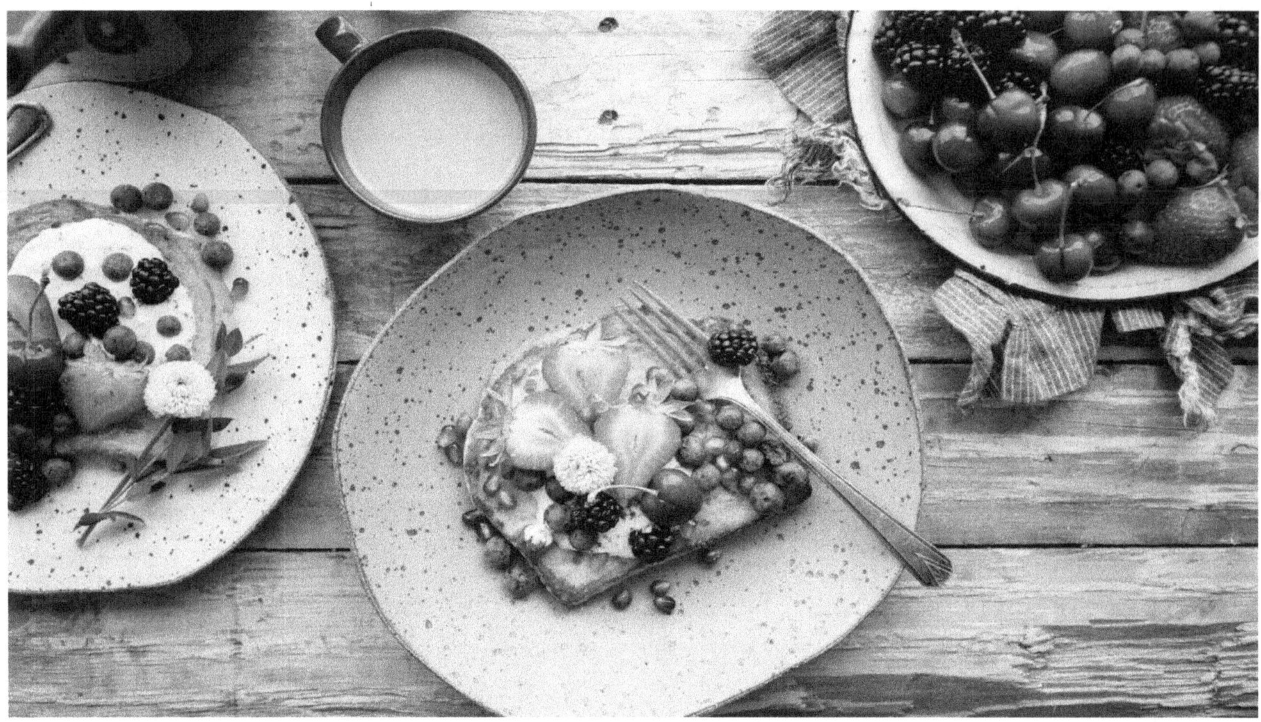

Sirtfoods are foods that contain sirtuins, which are also known as sirt proteins. These proteins help to regulate your cellular health. By activating certain organic groups in your body, a group of enzymes that work with NAD+ (nicotinamide adenine do nucleotide) will help you remove acetyl groups from proteins.

These activators are also minerals that help to restrict the calories you take in every day. Restricting your calorie intake will help you ward off issues tied to a rapid increase in weight. Another thing these minerals do is to treat various age-related diseases. The Sirtfood Diet is the better approach to move weight rapidly without extremist dieting by actuating the equivalent 'skinny gene' pathways usually initiated by exercise and fasting. Certain nourishments contain synthetic compounds called polyphenols that put mellow weight on our phones, turning on genes that imitate the impacts of fasting and exercise.

Add sound Sirtfoods to your diet for successful and supported weight reduction, mind-blowing energy, and gleaming well-being. Switch on your muscle to fat ratio's consuming forces, supercharge weight reduction, and help fight off infection with this simple-to-follow diet created by the specialists in healthful medication who demonstrated the effect of Sirtfoods. Dim chocolate, espresso, kale – these are altogether nourishments that enact sirtuins and switch on the alleged 'skinny gene' pathways in the body.

The Sirtfood Diet gives you a primary, reliable eating method for weight reduction, tasty simple to-make plans, and a support plan for delayed achievement. It is a diet of consideration, not avoidance, and Sirtfoods are broadly accessible and reasonable. This diet urges you to get your blade and fork and appreciate eating flavorful solid food while seeing the well-being and weight reduction benefits.

Sources of Sirtuin Proteins

You can get sirtuin proteins from all plants. Sirtuin proteins are highly concentrated in natural plant compounds. However, in fruits and vegetables, it is found in a smaller proportion. The ones that have the sirtuin proteins include:

1. Onions

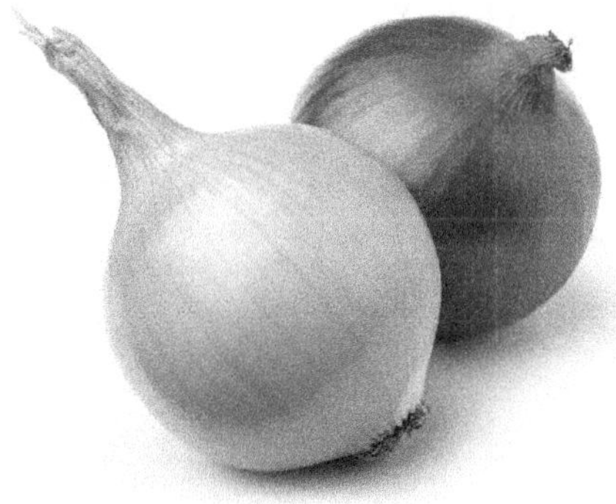

2. Kale

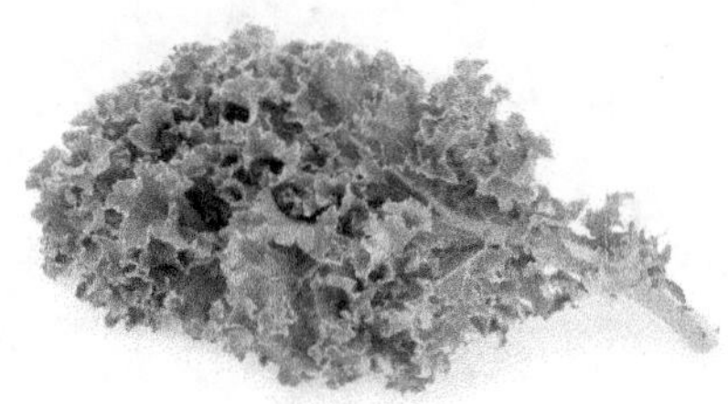

3. **Cocoa powder**

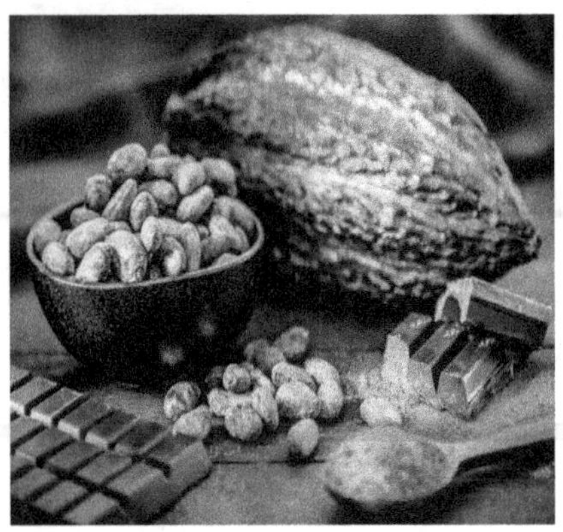

4. **Parsley**

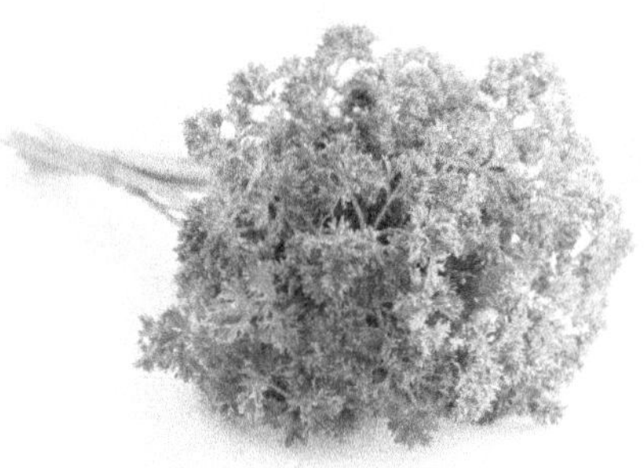

5. **Indian spice**

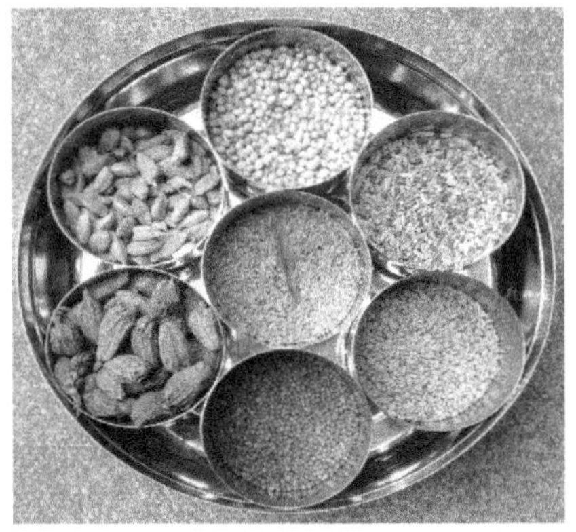

6. Turmeric

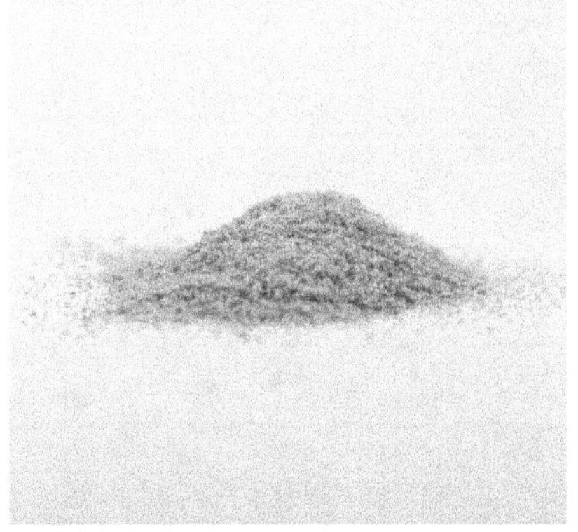

7. Green tea

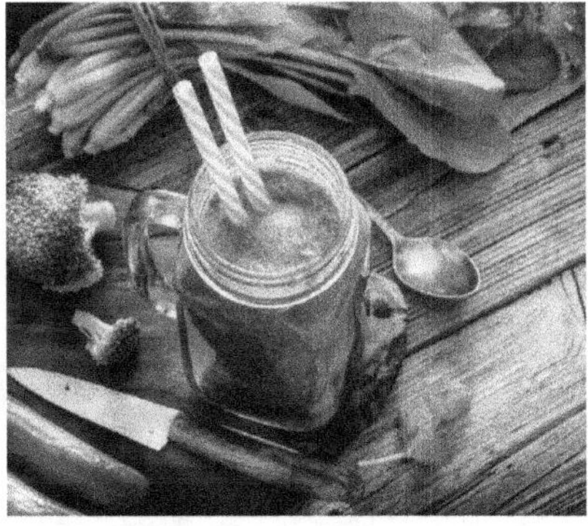

The sirtuin proteins in the food items listed above will help to preserve your muscles, which occur when the proteins trigger metabolism within your cells, which is done by following procedures such as extreme calorie restriction and extreme exercises, which are done to assist the proteins in burning the fat in your body.

Other food items that contain sirtuins include:

1. Arugula

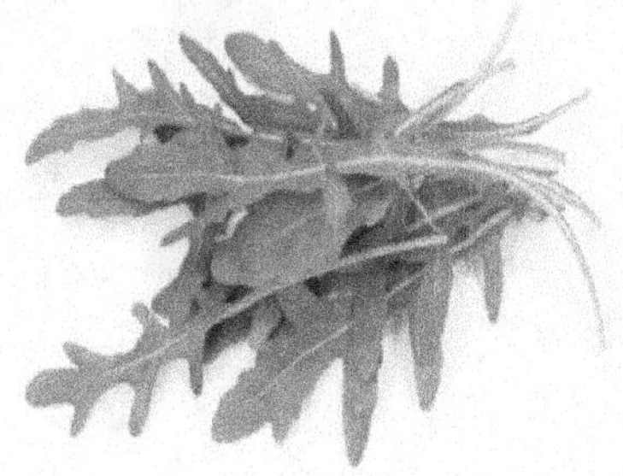

2. Buckwheat

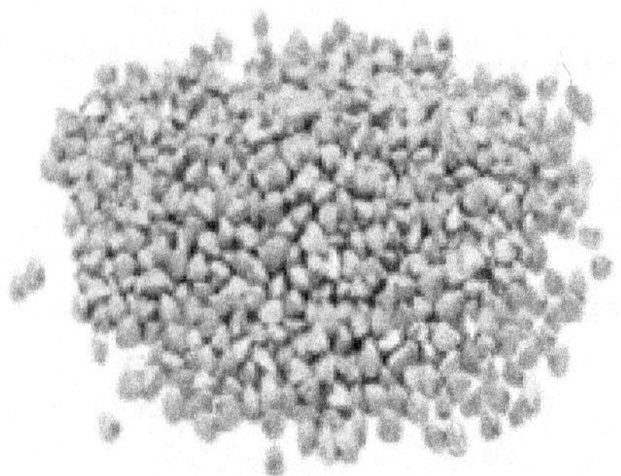

3. Celery

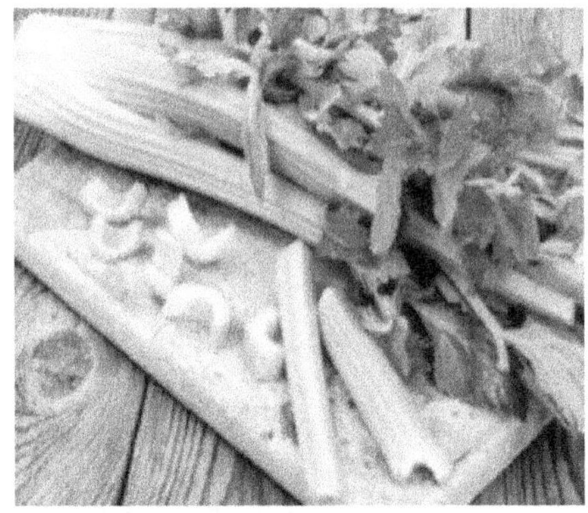

4. Capers

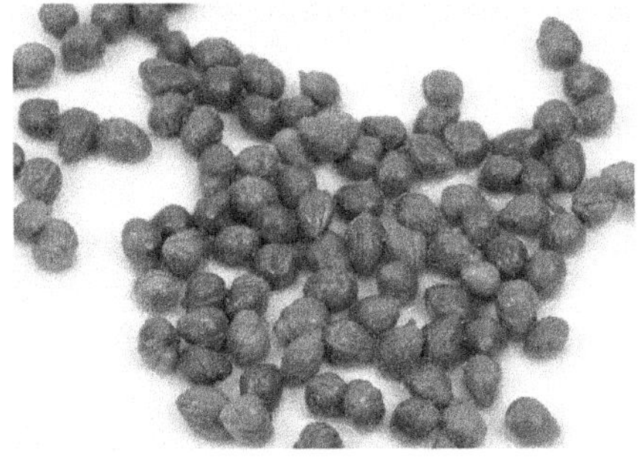

5. Chili pepper

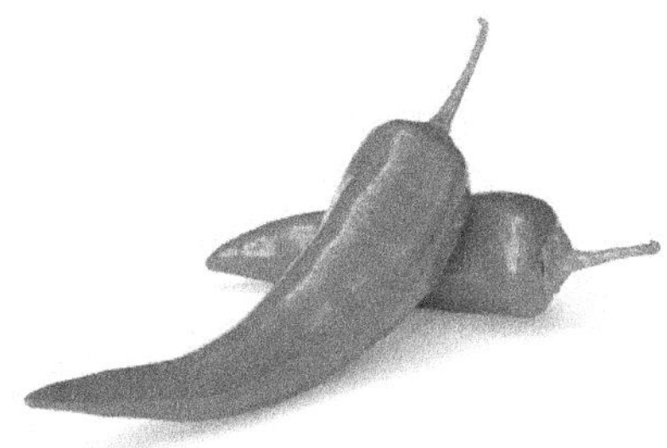

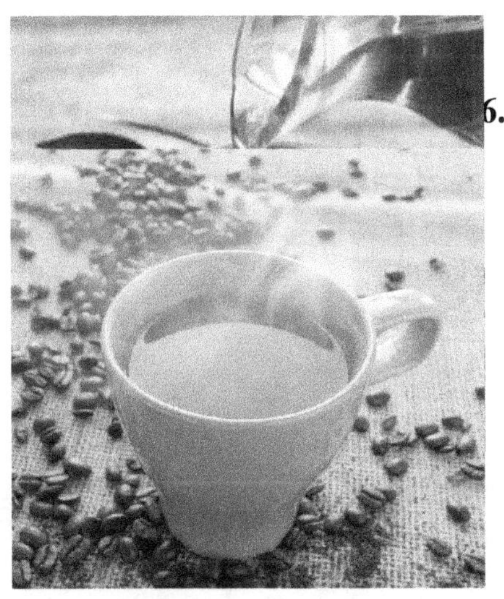

6. Coffee

7. Extra virgin oil

8. Garlic

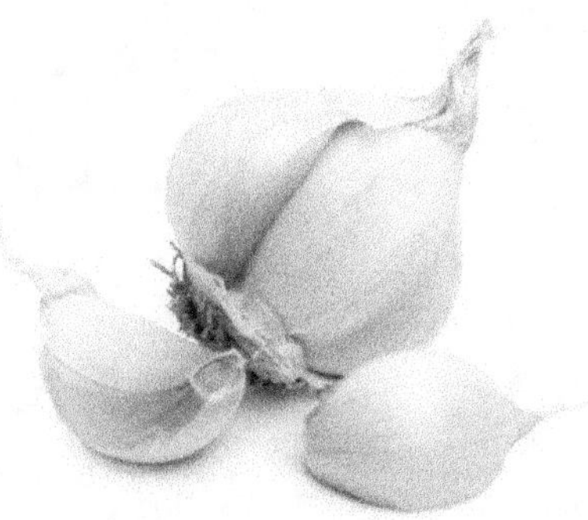

9. Strawberries

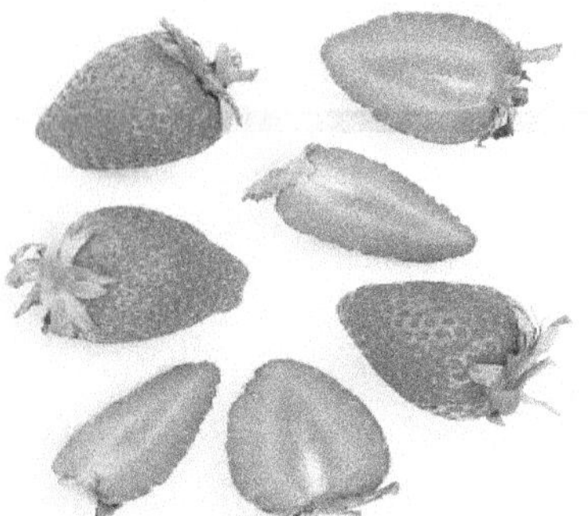

10. Soybeans

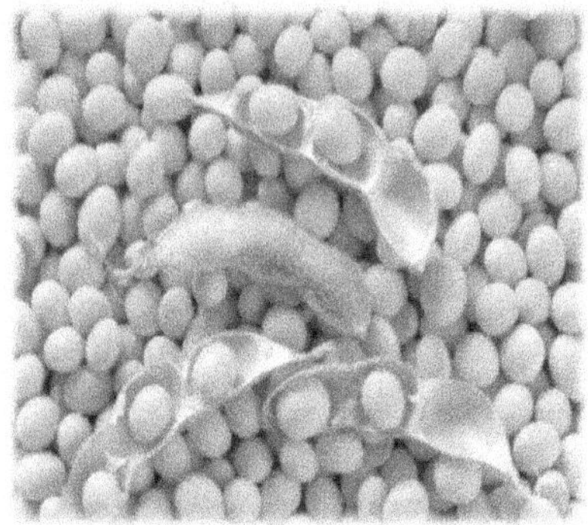

11. Matcha green tea

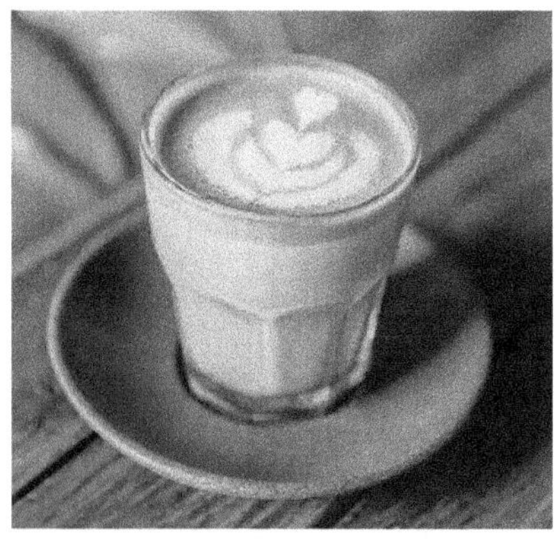

12. Walnuts

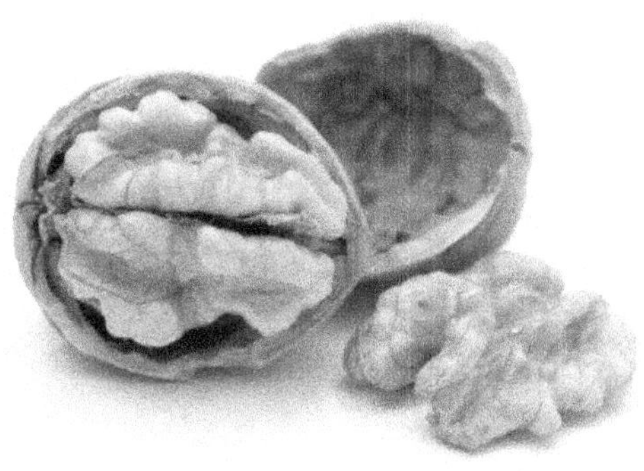

13. Bird's eye chilli

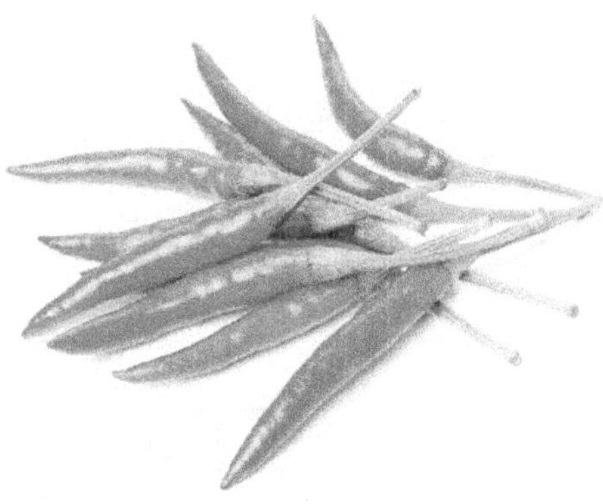

14. Medjool dates

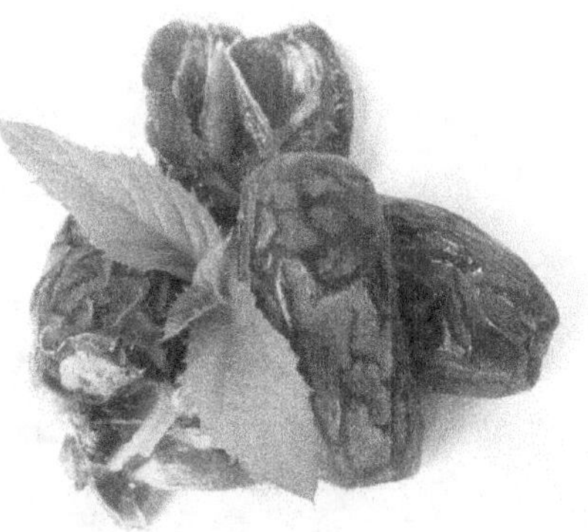

15. Red chicory

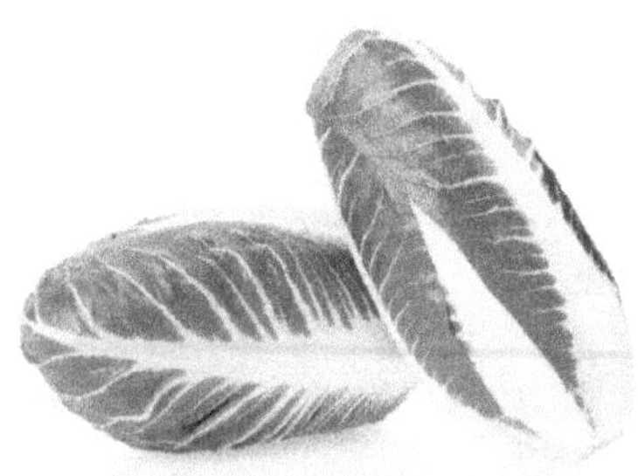

16. Blueberries

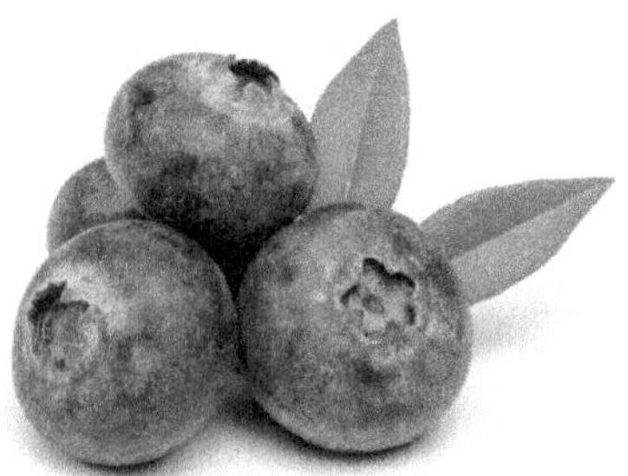

The activating compounds in the food items include; quercetin, kaempferol, curcumin, Apigenin, and epigallocatechin Gallate. With these, you can lose seven pounds of weight in seven days without losing your muscle mass!

How It works

The diet has two simple-to-follow phases:

Phase 1. This goes on for seven days.

Phase 2. This 14-day upkeep is planned to assist you with getting in shape consistently. You can eat three adjusted sirtfood-rich suppers always, in addition to one green juice.

The two phases can be rehashed at whatever point you like for fat-misfortune support.

What occurs after the subsequent phase? What's more, is this sort of diet genuinely reasonable?

The possibility of "sirtifying" suppers is for the individuals who have finished Phases 1 and 2 yet, at the same time, need to proceed in the Sirtfood way. It includes taking your number one dish and giving it a Sirtfood bend. Plans incorporate ordinary top picks like chicken curry, bean stew con-Carne, pizza, and flapjacks.

The Sirtfood Diet isn't intended to be a coincidental 'diet' yet rather a lifestyle. You are energized, whenever you've finished the initial three weeks, to keep eating a diet wealthy in Sirtfoods and to keep drinking your day by day green juice. There are currently numerous Sirtfood Diet formula books accessible, with plans for more Sirtfood-rich fundamental dinners, as well as plans for options in contrast to the green juice. There are even a few plans for Sirtfood pastries. These books also include more clues and tips for following the Sirtfood Diet. Phases 1 and 2 can be rehashed as and when fundamental for well-being support or if things have gone off track.

How To Start

Day by day, squeezes are fundamental to the Sirtfood Diet, so ensure you have a juicer. You'll additionally require three essential ingredients.

Matcha is a powdered green tea and a significant fixing in the green juices. It's promptly accessible on the web if your neighborhood well-being food shop doesn't stock it. Also, lovage – a spice in the green juice formula – which can be quite hard to track down. In any case, it's anything but complicated to purchase seeds online to develop it in a pot on a windowsill. Last is buckwheat. It's a fabulous option in contrast to more normal grains. However, most markets blend buckwheat and wheat in their items. You're bound to discover 100% buckwheat items in your nearby well-being food store.

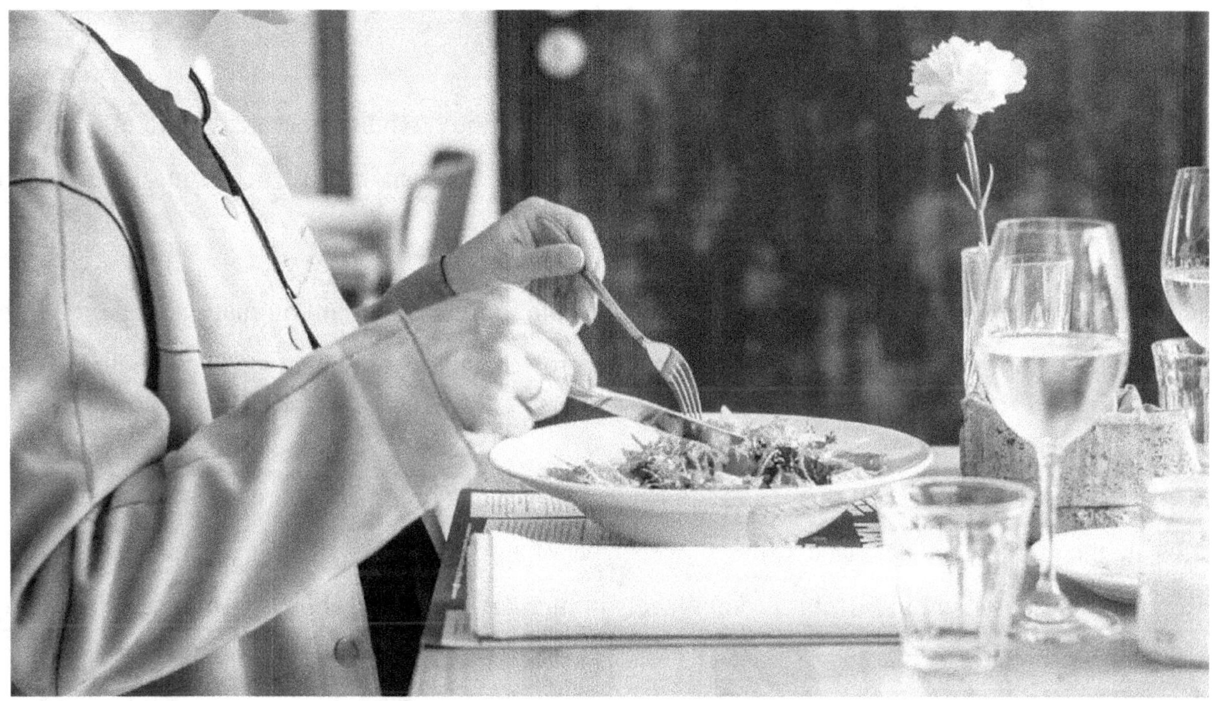

According to nutritionist Rob Hobson, Sirtfoods means foods high in Sirtuins activators. Sirtuins help to protect the body cells from damaging, getting inflamed, and dying through sickness and disease. Scientific research has also proven that they also work to enhance the body muscle, regulate metabolic rate, and also burn fat.

Is Sirtfoods The Revolutionary Superfoods?

It's not a mere say that Sirtfoods is lovely and suitable for everyone. They are high in nutrients and packed with healthy compounds and properties.

Few studies have been able to recommend that Sirtfoods have lots of healthy benefits. For instance, consuming the right amount of dark chocolate rich in cocoa content tends to minimize the risk of heart disease and help get rid of inflammation. Also, green tea is very potent in combating the risk of stroke and even all types of diabetes and likewise effective in lowering blood pressure. Additionally, turmeric is high in anti-inflammatory properties and well packed with high beneficiary effects on the body and can guide the body against all forms of health-related conditions. Most Sirtfoods have proven to have significant beneficiary effects in humans.

There seems to be no concrete evidence on the beneficiary effects of an increased level of sirtuin proteins in humans. But particular research in cell lines and other animals has proven to be beneficial. For instance, an increase in the level of a certain Sirtuins protein level leads to prolonged lifespan in worms, yeast, and mice.

In the process of calorie restriction, sirtuin proteins notify the body to burn more fat to gain more energy and enhance insulin sensitivity. A particular study in mice stated that an increase in Sirtuins levels results in fat loss.

Other evidence also suggests that Sirtuins plays a vital role in minimizing inflammation, preventing the growth and development of tumors, and reducing the growth and development of heart-related disease and Alzheimer's.

Studies in humans and mice cell lines have indicated positive outcomes, but there are no human studies yet to state the impact that increased Sirtuins levels have on humans. Thus, there is no concrete evidence to ascertain that increment in Sirtuins protein levels in humans will bring about a prolonged lifespan or reduce the risk of cancer.

There's on-going research on the development of compounds that will be potent at increasing Sirtuins protein levels in the human body. Due to this, studies are continuing to know the impacts of Sirtuins in the human body.

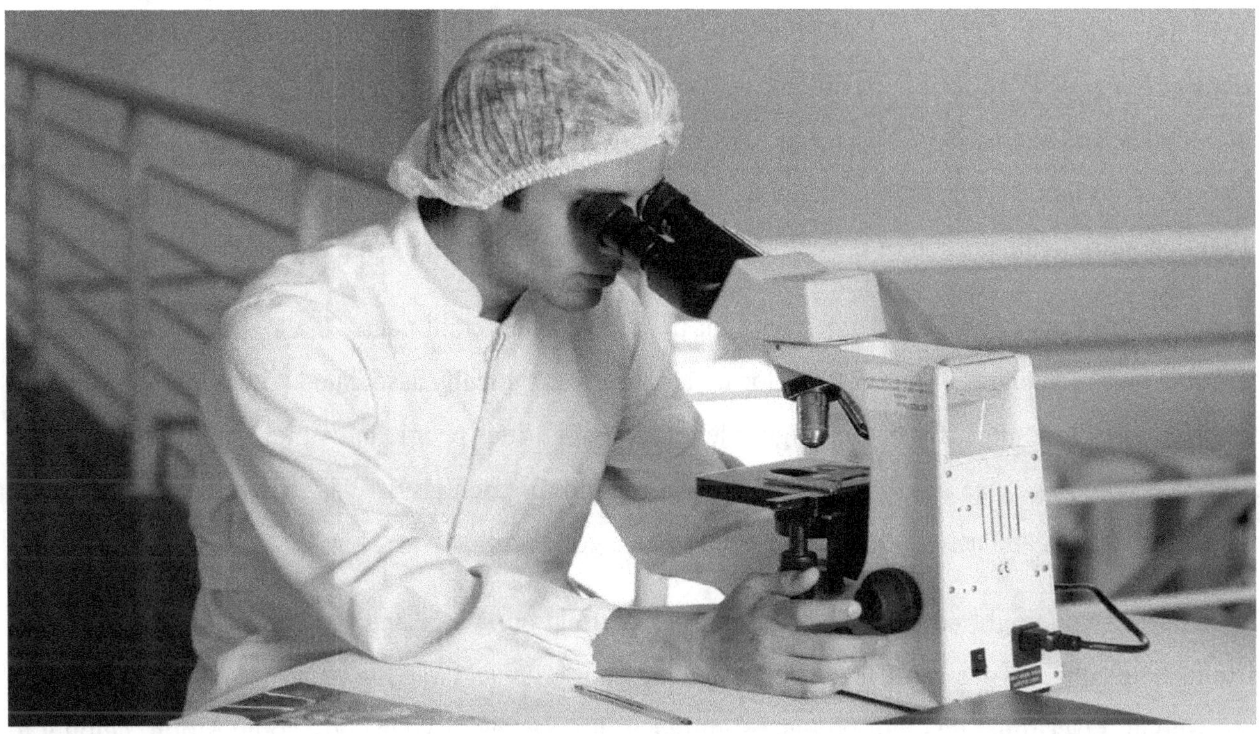

Did you know that thousands of people have unlocked incredible and aesthetic physiques by following the sirtfood diet?

The primary lean gene, also known as a sirtuin, on which this dieting style got its name, was first found in 1984, not in humans but yeasts. Polyphenol is a well-known chemical compound present in the body. It acts on an essential lean gene to activate and perform fat-burning blits inside the human body. To be very specific, sirtfoods are those which contain high levels of a chemical compound called polyphenol. This compound is not uniformly distributed in sirtfoods, but every sirtfood contains particular amounts of polyphenols.

Polyphenols are the compounds that are present naturally in sirtfoods, and many types of research conducted on these foods have confirmed that these foods have the highest impacts when losing extra pounds of fats from the body. Polyphenols are essential precursors in the fat burning cycle of the body called lipolysis. Free fatty acids in our blood are subjected to digestion and then excretion from the body through the lipase enzyme. Foods rich in Polyphenols cause much increase in lipase enzyme levels and thus more fat burning blits in the body.

Fighting Fat

There are mainly two types of body Fat - the white adipose tissue and brown adipose tissue. **_White adipose tissue, or WAT_** as it is commonly abbreviated, is the fat made for storage. It's where your spare energy goes, and having more WAT makes it easier to store and gain fat. **_Brown adipose tissue, or BAT_**, is a type of fat tissue typically associated with burning fat. BAT helps us warm and contains high levels of mitochondria – the portion of the cell that is responsible for producing energy.

Leaner people have higher levels of brown fat than their overweight peers. BAT is located around the neck and back. In contrast, your WAT is located in the areas typically associated with obesity – your gut, buttocks, chest, and hips. By having higher levels of BAT, fitter people have more ability to shake off calories through exercise and thermal release, so although research on BAT is still in its nascent stages, higher BAT levels and activity is hypothesized to be a good thing.

Of course, as you might now anticipate, sirtuins also affect our WAT and BAT levels. More precisely, sirtuins help convert your WAT into BAT, changing your body and making it easier to burn calories and lose weight. Over time, this will produce significant differences in your body composition, helping to make you lose weight and become lean.

The foods to be introduced into the Sirt Diet are, for example, meat, fish, kale, chocolate, red wine, olive oil. It is not necessary to reduce the portion quantities; on the contrary, the results are obtained by eating abundantly. The fat deposits on the body sometimes grow faster than we would like. Fasting alone doesn't get them away. There is only one way to get rid of the excess energy: more exercise.

Chocolate and Wine

Red wine and dark chocolate are the foods that are a big "YES" for the Americans. It is no less than good news for them that these two foods along with some others, fall in the list of sirtfoods that can help them to achieve their dream weight. These foods contain polyphenols that are nothing but naturally occurring chemicals that essentially activate the skinny gene and help to mimic whatever efforts you put into doing exercise and fasting. The foods that also fall in this list include olive oil, parsley, Medjool dates, matcha green tea, kale, soy, strawberries, onion, buckwheat, walnuts, lovage, red chicory, capers, turmeric, arugula, blueberries, and coffee.

These foods trigger the body to produce sirtuins at higher levels. This diet has been introduced as the new revolutionary diet that is essential for activating this gene that has many roles to play in your body. From regulating various functions to reducing inflammation and increasing lifespan, they are considered as vital genes that are very important.

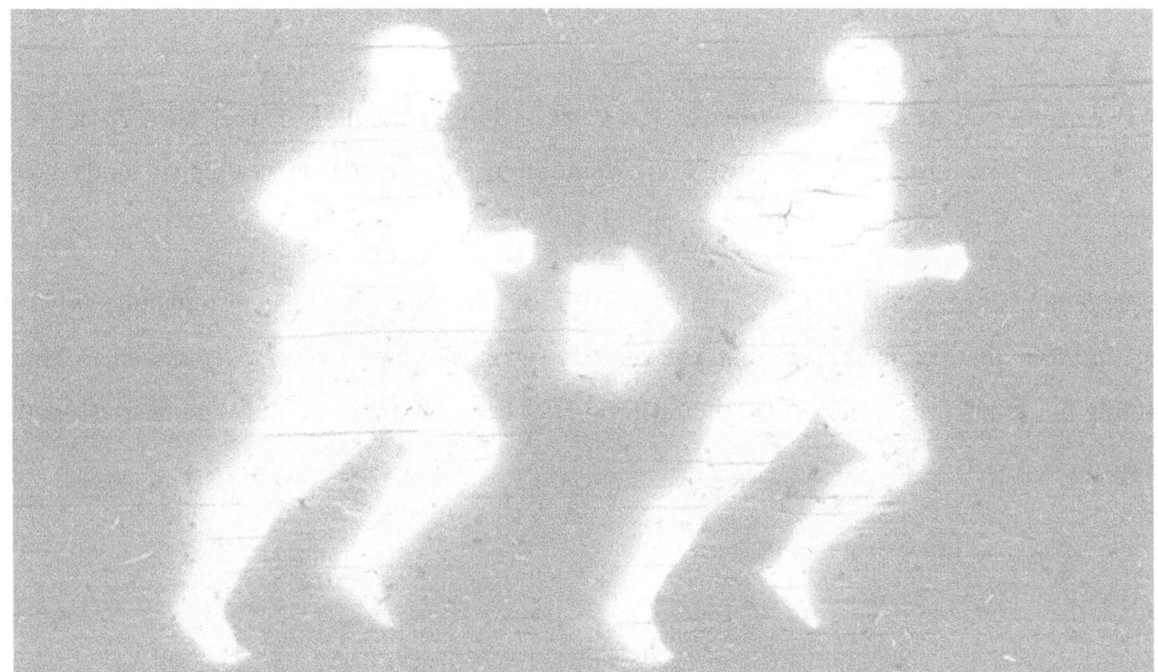

This diet is certainly not for everyone, and it requires a lot of funds and energy to get through the meal preparation. The book includes several recipes about halfway through your reading, but many of the ingredients are so special that consumers found it hard to find them at the grocery store, as well as the tastes were so different in the beginning. Generally, this diet is backed by science, as many case studies have been shown, but for the average person, the possibility of seeing results from this diet may be a long shot. Just remember; the greater the effort, the sweeter the reward. The Sirt Diet program will detoxify your body for seven days, and then you'll need to keep eating sirtfoods to see the weight coming off and stop your body from getting it all back.

This program includes two phases:

Phase 1

This process will limit you to 1,000 calories a day for a week, and two of your meals will be green drinks rich in Sirtfoods such as lettuce, celery, parsley, green tea, and lemon. Even rich in Sirtfoods like beef, chicken, spinach, or buckwheat noodles, you can have one meal per day.

You are permitted to increase the caloric intake to 1,500 calories during this process, and you are still consuming the two green drinks, but you are now permitted to add another meal to the day, allowing two meals and two beverages. This phase can last up to 14 days.

After The Diet

Those two stages may be repeated as often as you wish for further weight loss. However, upon finishing those stages, you are advised to start "sirtifying" your diet by consistently integrating sirtfoods into your meals.

There are a number of Sirtfood Diet books that are full of rich recipes. You can also include sirtfoods as a snack in your diet, or in recipes that you already have. You are further encouraged to continue consuming the green juice daily. Thus, the Sirtfood Diet becomes more of a change in lifestyle than a one-time diet.

Green Juice and Sirt Food

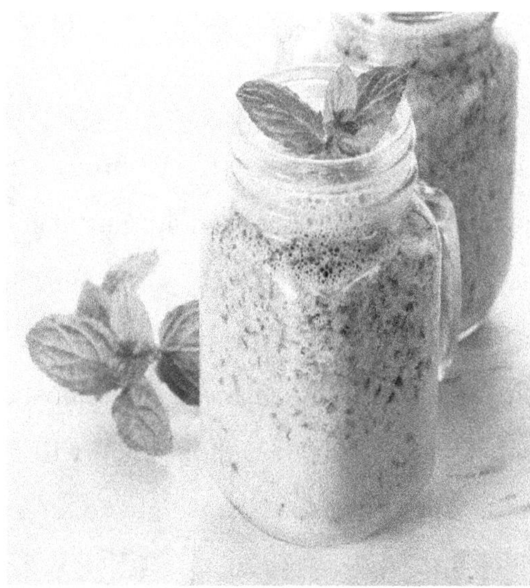

The sirtfood diet requires drinking two to three green juices every day. It is a completely natural juice and characterized by its green color given by its ingredients. This drink has the greatest ability to purify and satiate. Juices during the diet should be consumed 1 hour before the solid meal or 2 hours after. Another rule is that you must have dinner by 7:00pm.

As we have seen, it is a diet that, above all in the first days, is based on a miraculous green juice. A completely natural drink that is combined first with one and then with two solid meals. This juice is an important part of the diet because it has the ability to cleanse and detoxify, and is the main character in the first week of the Sirt program. You have to prepare it three times a day and you will need a centrifuge and a kitchen scale, because the ingredients are listed by weight. The recipe is below:

Ingredients:

75g of curly kale

30g of rocket

5g of parsley

150g of green celery with leaves

½ green apple

½ lemon juice

½ teaspoon matcha tea

Directions:

Centrifuge kale, rocket and parsley.

Add grated celery and apple; enrich with half a squeezed lemon and half a teaspoon of matcha tea.

Drink immediately so you don't miss out on the valuable benefits of nutrients.

The Third Phase, a Blessing Forever

You may repeat the two phases as often as you would like to meet your weight loss goals. Even if you have achieved it, the creators of the diet suggest adopting sirtfoods for your day-to-day needs because they have designed this diet as an alternative way of living.

Resume Your Workout Routines

Since your calorie limit for the first couple of weeks into the diet, it is best to either lessen or stop working out while your body gets used to its new condition. No two persons are exactly alike, so the best thing you can do to know when you can start exercising like you usually do it by paying closer attention to your body.

To be on the safer side of things, most followers opt to resume their regular workout schedule after clearing phase 2 of the diet. By then, you would feel more energized, and more capable of completing your usual exercise sets.

Take note that even though a sirtfood diet does not require you to exercise to unlock its benefits, it would still be best for the overall wellness of your body and mind to remain fit and active every day.

Try Out Sirtfood Smoothies With Protein Powder

If you decide to start exercising again, you should add smoothies that contain lots of sirtfoods and protein powder to help you reduce the soreness of your muscles, and keep you well energized throughout and after your workout.

Recipes for fun and tasty sirtfood smoothies can easily be found in blogs and recipe books dedicated to the Sirtfood Diet. If you are pretty confident with your skills in the kitchen, then feel free to experiment with the recommended ingredients, and discover the perfect smoothie combinations for your taste buds.

Invite Your Family and Friends to Try Out the Diet

One of the best ways to maintain your healthier diet is by getting the people around you involved in it as well. Studies show that the kind of company you keep can have a huge influence on your lifestyle, including what and how you eat. Let them also read this guide so that they will have a better idea of what it is, what it can do for them, and how they should go about it.

Consider adopting the principles of the Sirtfood Diet as part of your way of life. It is just not a one-time, quick-fix meal plan, and you cannot go wrong by adding more sirtfoods into your day-to-day diet.

Do I exercise during phase 1?

Regular exercise is one of the best things you can do for your health, and doing some moderate exercise can improve your diet's weight loss and wellbeing. As a general rule, during the sirtfood diet's first seven days, we advise you to maintain your normal level of exercise and physical activity.

I am slim — can I follow the diet?

For anyone who is underweight, we do not recommend phase 1 of the sirtfood diet. Calculating your body mass index or bmi is a safe way to nd it out if you are underweight. You can easily calculate this by using one of the numerous online bmi calculators, as long as you know your height and weight. If your bmi is 18.5 or less, we do not suggest embarking on a diet phase 1. We would also advise caution if your bmi is between 18.5 and 20 because following the diet can mean that your bmi falls below 18.5. While many people strive to be super-skinny, the fact is that underweight may have a detrimental effect on many health factors, leading to a lower immune system, an increased risk of osteoporosis (weakening bones), and fertility issues. Though phase 1 of the diet is not recommended if you are underweight, we also promote the incorporation of plenty of sirtfoods into a healthy way of eating so that all the health benefits of these foods can be obtained.

If you're slim but have a good range of bmi (20–25), however, there's absolutely nothing to stop you from getting started. A majority of the pilot trial participants had bmis in the healthy range, but still lost impressive amounts of weight and got more toned. Importantly, many registered a significant increase in strength, vitality, and appearance levels. Mind that the sirtfood diet is about health promotion, as well as weight loss.

I am obese — is sirtfood correct for me?

Hey! Don't be put off by the fact that only a tiny number of our pilot study participants were obese. That is because the pilot research was performed in a fitness and fitness community, where participants are usually more health-conscious and tighter. Instead, be motivated by the fact that the few who were obese had much better outcomes than our participants who were healthy-weight. The thousands of people who tried the diet in the real world repeated those findings. You will also expect to reap the greatest improvements in your well-being, based on the research into sirtuin activation. Being obese increases the risk of many chronic health problems, yet these are the very illnesses against which sirtfoods helps to protect.

I reached my target weight, and don't want to lose any more — do I stop sirtfoods eating?

First of all, congratulations on your success in terms of weight loss! With sirtfoods, you've had great success, but it doesn't stop now. While we do not recommend further restriction on calories, your diet should still provide ample sirtfood. Most of our customers are now at their optimal body composition but continue to consume diets high in sirtfood. The great thing about sirtfoods is they are a lifestyle. In terms of weight control, the best way to think of them is that they help get the body to the weight and shape it was meant to be. They work from here to sustain and keep you looking fantastic and feeling great. Ultimately, this is the aim we wish for all followers of the sirtfood diet.

I've finished phase 2—do I now drink the sirtfood green juice in the morning?

The green juice is our favorite way to start the day with a great hit from sirtfoods, so we support its long-term consumption. Our sirtfood green juice has been carefully designed to include ingredients that provide a full spectrum of sirtuin-activating nutrients in effective dose-boosting fat-burning and wellness. We 're all about variety, however, and while we suggest that you start with a morning juice, we completely support anyone wanting to play with various sirtfood juice concoctions.

I take medication — is it still okay to follow the diet?

The sirtfood diet is ideal for most people, but due to its powerful effects on fat burning and wellbeing, it can alter the processes of certain diseases and the drug acts recommended by your doctor. Similarly, other drugs are not appropriate in a state of fasting.

During the sirtfood diet trial, we assessed each individual's suitability before they embarked on the diet , especially those taking medication. Clearly, we can't do it for you, but if you suffer from a significant health condition, take prescription medications, or have any reasons to think about going on a diet, we recommend that you speak to your doctor about it. The chances for you are it will be a fine and indeed profound benefit, but it is necessary to test.

Should I adopt the diet if I am pregnant?

If you are trying to conceive or are pregnant or breastfeeding, we do not suggest embarking on the sirtfood diet. It is a powerful diet for weight loss, which makes it inappropriate. Don't be put off eating plenty of sirtfoods, though, as these are incredibly nutritious foods to be consumed as part of a balanced and varied pregnancy diet. Because of its alcohol content, you will want to avoid red wine and limit caffeinated items such as coffee, green tea, and cocoa to not exceed 200 milligrams of caffeine per day during pregnancy (one mug of instant coffee typically contains about 100 milligrams of caffeine). Recommendations do not exceed four cups of green tea a day and do avoid matcha altogether. Other than that, the benefits of having sirtfoods in your diet are free to reap.

Are sirtfoods suitable for children?

The sirtfood diet is a strong diet for weight loss and not intended for kids, though that doesn't mean that kids will miss out on the excellent health benefits provided by adding more sirtfoods to their overall diet.

Do I take any supplements?

Unless your doctor or other health care professional has specifically prescribed for you, we do not recommend indiscriminate use of nutritional supplements. You will be ingesting from sirtfoods a large and synergistic variety of natural plant compounds, and it is these that will do you good. You can't reproduce these benefits with nutritional supplements, and in fact, some nutritional supplements like antioxidants, particularly if taken at high doses, can actually interfere with sirtfood's beneficial effects, which is the last thing you want.

Whenever possible, we think that having the nutrients you need from consuming a healthy diet rich in sirtfoods is much easier than taking the nutrients in the form of a tablet. However, vegans will have different dietary requirements, and our detailed guidelines can be found on pages 131–132 for those adopting strictly plant-based diets. Furthermore, because plant proteins are lower in leucine, the amino acid that enhances sirtfoods' behavior, we have found that vegans can benefit from supplementing their diet with effective vegan protein powder. This refers in particular to those who perform high levels of exercise. This supplement will be taken off the sirtfood green juice at a different time of day.

How can I repeat phases 1 and 2?

You can repeat phase 1 again if you feel you need a weight-loss or a health boost. To ensure long-term adverse effects of calorie restriction on your metabolism are not present, you should wait at least a month before returning. However, we find that most people need to repeat it no more frequently than at most once every three months and keep getting amazing results. Instead, if you have gone off course, need some fine-tuning, or want a little more sirtfood pressure, we suggest that you repeat as much as you want any or all of the phase 2 days. Phase 2 is, after all, about developing a lifelong way to feed. Remember, the sirtfood diet's beauty is that it doesn't require you to feel like you're endlessly on a diet, but rather it's the springboard to develop positive lifelong dietary changes that create a lighter, leaner, healthier you.

Does the sirtfood diet have enough fiber?

Naturally, a lot of sirtfoods are rich in fiber. Onions, endive, and walnuts are notable sources, with buckwheat and medjool dates really standing out, meaning the fiber department is not short of a sirtfood-rich diet. Even during phase 1, when food consumption is reduced, most of us will still consume a fiber quantity that we are used to, particularly if we select from the menu options the recipes that contain buckwheat, beans, and lentils. However, for others known to be susceptible to intestinal problems such as constipation without higher fiber intakes, a suitable fiber supplement may be considered during phase 1, especially days 1 to 3, which should be discussed with your health care professional.

I've read about superfoods — should I include these in my diet too?

The first thing you need to know about the term superfood is that it's a marketing slogan, not a scientific term at all. You don't need to worry about so-called superfoods because the sirtfood diet brings together the planet's healthiest foods into a revolutionary new way of eating. Just as relying on a simple vitamin pill to make us safe is a mistake, so relying on a single superfood to do the same is also a mistake. It is the entire diet, consisting of a wide spectrum of sirtfoods and their vast array of natural compounds, acting in synergy, which is the true secret to achieving weight loss and lifelong health.

Do I need to do phase 1 for seven days?

There is nothing special about seven days in phase 1. Simply this is what we agreed for our case. We opted for that because it was long enough to produce good results, but not long enough to make it arduous. It also blends seamlessly into the lives of men. It was tested for seven days and what is known to be successful. However, if you need to cut it short by a day or two for whatever reason, do so by completing until the end of day 5 or day 6. Don't worry, the lion's share of the benefits will still be reaped.

Can I eat what I want once I eat plenty of sirtfoods and results still show?

One of the main reasons why the sirtfood diet works so well in the long term is that it encourages good food rather than demonizing poor food. Exclusion diets just aren't effective long-term. It is true that processed foods high in sugars and fats decrease sirtuin activity in the body, thus reducing the benefits of sirtfoods by high consumption. However, if you keep your attention on eating a diet rich in sirtfoods, you will end up consuming much less garbage than the average person as a result if you are happily fulfilled and have less appetite for certain refined foods. If you sometimes indulge in these refined foods, don't worry about it — the strength of sirtfoods, the rest of the time, will ensure that you are still reaping the benefits.

Can I eat as many non-sirtfoods, after eating the sirtfoods as I want and still lose weight?

Hey! Note, calories and the urge to count them are a modern-day "advancement." Such an idea did not exist through societies and countless generations since there was simply no need. People ate as they felt like it and remained slim and disease-free. Given the impact of sirtfoods on metabolism and appetite control, you just don't have to worry about eating too many of these. Although this is not an invitation to an all-you-can-eat contest, feel free to consume as much sirtfood as your natural appetite can fulfill.

Our only exception is medjool dates. Their presence reveals how high-sugar foods should not be bad for you when consumed in the intended form of nature, and in moderation. However, moderation is key to making dates an indulgent treat with no guilt. As for alcohol, when it comes to the consumption of red wine, it goes without saying that it should be consumed responsibly and safely under the guidelines of the government.

Are they organic?

We will urge you to a perfect world to opt for organic produce whenever possible, practical, and affordable. While there is no evidence that the levels of traditional vitamins and minerals differ from organic to non-organic, what about the nutrients that activate sirtuin?

Organic produce is likely to carry a richer content of sirtuin-activating nutrients. Note that the sirtuin-activating polyphenols present in plant foods are developed in response to environmental stresses, and without the heavy use of pesticides, organically grown crops would have to fight that much harder to discourage and prevent predators of the environment. This is likely to result in higher levels of polyphenols being generated, potentially making organic sirtfood more potent than its non-organic counterpart. While organic is preferable, if you opt for non-organic produce, you will still get great results from the sirtfood diet. Green, on top, is just the cherry.

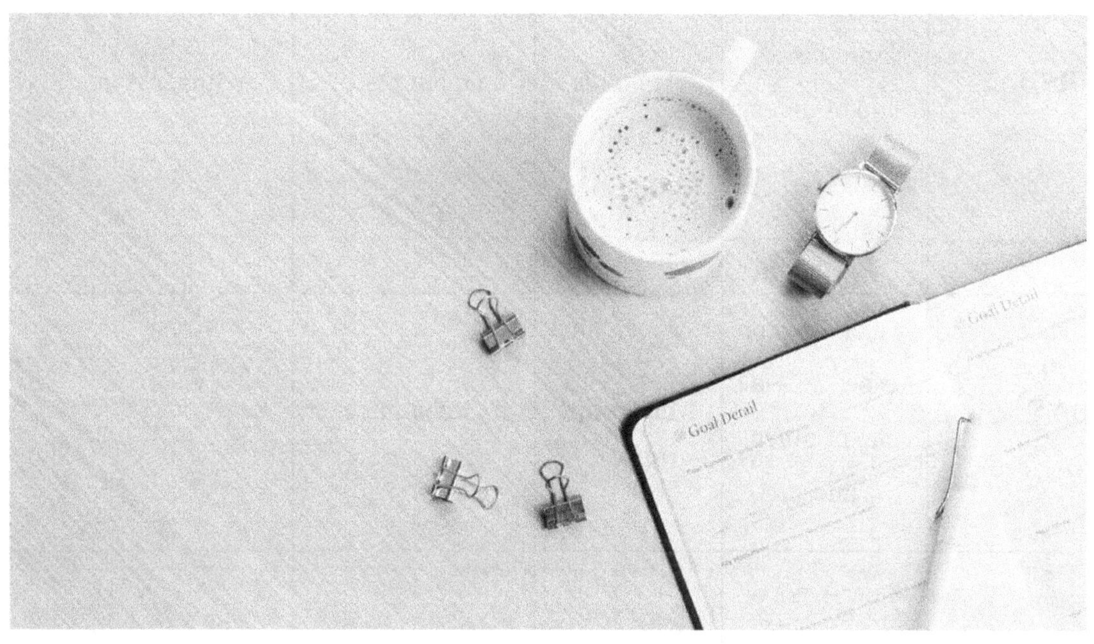

DAY	BREAKFAST	LUNCH	SNACK	DINNER
PHASE 1				
MONDAY	water + tea or espresso + a cup of green juice;	2 Green juices	A square of dark chocolate	Shrimp and Endives
TUESDAY	water + tea or espresso + a cup of green juice;	2 Green juices	A square of dark chocolate	Tuna and Tomatoes
WEDNESDAY	water + tea or espresso + a cup of green juice;	2 Green juices	A square of dark chocolate	Wow Cola Chicken
PHASE 2				

THURSDAY	water + tea or espresso + a cup of green juice;	Scallops with Almonds and Mushrooms	Green juice	Ginger Asian Slaw
FRIDAY	water + tea or espresso + a cup of green juice;	Tofu Mushroom Soup	Green juice	
SATURDAY	water + tea or espresso + a cup of green juice;	Pork with pak choi	Green juice	Stuffed Mushrooms
SUNDAY	water + tea or espresso + a cup of green juice;	Cherry Chicken Lettuce Wraps	Green juice	Herring Cold Meat Salad

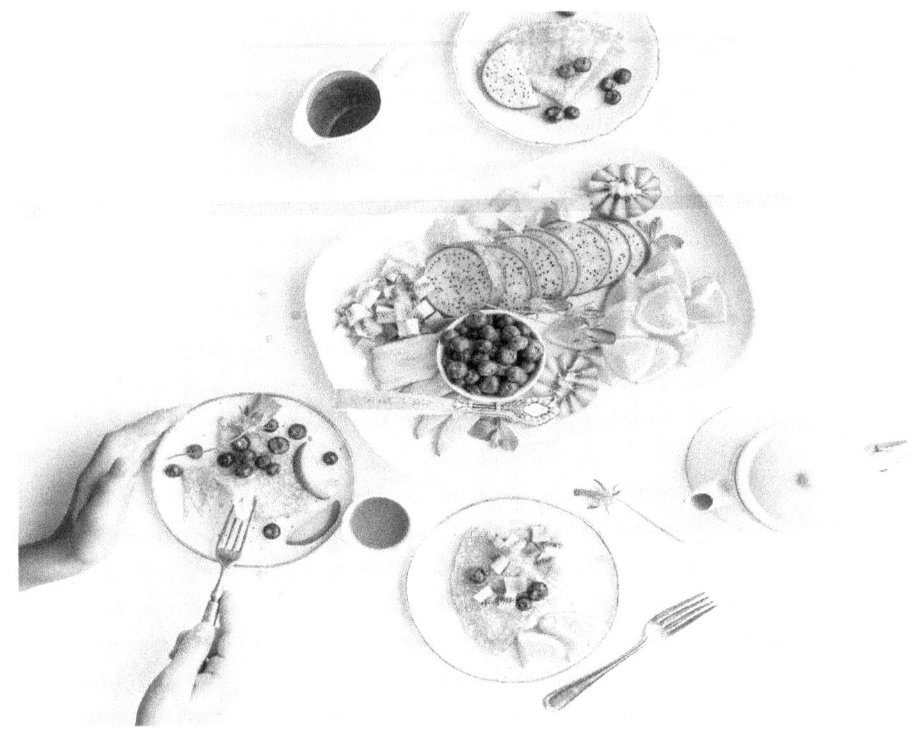

1. Vegetable Hash with White Beans

Preparation Time: 15 Minutes

Cooking Time: 23 Minutes

Servings: 4

Ingredients:

1 leek (white part only), finely chopped

1 red bell pepper, deseeded and diced

Water, as needed

2 teaspoons of rosemary, minced

3 cloves garlic, peeled and minced

1 medium sweet potato, peeled and diced

1 large turnip, peeled and diced

2 cups cooked white beans, or 1 (15-ounce / 425-g) can drain and rinse

1 orange, juice and zest

1 cup chopped kale

Salt, to taste (optional)

Freshly ground black pepper, to taste

Directions:

Put the leek and red pepper in a large saucepan over medium heat and sauté for 8 minutes, stirring occasionally. Add water, 1 to 3 tablespoons at a time, to keep them from sticking to the bottom of the pan.

Stir in the rosemary and garlic and sauté for 1 minute more.

Add the sweet potato, turnip, beans, and orange juice and zest, and stir well—heat until the vegetables are softened.

Add the kale and sprinkle with salt (if desired) and pepper. Cook for about 5 minutes or more until the kale is wilted.

Serve on a plate.

Nutrition: Calories: 245, Fat: 0.6g, Carbs: 48g, Protein: 11g

2. Ratatouille

Preparation Time: 20 Minutes

Cooking Time: 25 Minutes

Servings: 4

Ingredients:

1 medium red onion, peeled and diced

Water, as needed

4 cloves garlic, peeled and minced

1 medium red bell pepper, without seeds and diced

1 small zucchini, diced

1 medium eggplant stemmed and diced

1 large tomato, diced

½ cup chopped basil

Salt, to taste (optional)

Freshly ground black pepper, to taste

Directions:

Put the onion in a medium saucepan over medium heat and sauté for 10 minutes, stirring occasionally, or until the onion is tender. Add water 1 to 3 tablespoons at a time to keep it from sticking.

Add the garlic, red pepper, zucchini, and eggplant and stir well. Lid the saucepan and cook for 12 to 15 minutes, stirring occasionally.

Mix in the tomatoes and basil, then sprinkle with salt (if desired) and pepper. Serve immediately.

Nutrition: Calories: 76, Fat: 1g, Carbs: 15g, Protein: 2g

3. Baingan Bharta (Indian Spiced Eggplant)

Preparation Time: 15 Minutes

Cooking Time: 25 Minutes

Servings: 4

Ingredents:

2 medium onions, peeled and diced

1 large red bell pepper, deseeded and diced

Water, as needed

2 large tomatoes, finely chopped

2 medium eggplants, stemmed, peeled, and cut into ½-inch dices

3 tablespoons of ginger, grated

1 teaspoon coriander seed, toasted and ground

2 teaspoons cumin seeds, toasted and ground

½ teaspoon crushed red pepper flakes

A pinch of cloves

Salt, to taste (optional)

½ bunch cilantro, leaves, and tender stems, finely sliced

Directions:

Combine the onions and red pepper in a large saucepan and cook over medium heat for about 10 to 12 minutes. Include water 1 to 2 tablespoons at the moment to keep them from sticking to the pan.

Stir in the tomatoes, eggplant, ginger, coriander, cumin, crushed red pepper flakes, and cloves and cook for just about 12 to 15 minutes, or until the vegetables are tender.

Sprinkle with the salt, if desired. Garnish with the cilantro and serve warm.

Nutrition: Calories: 140, Fat: 1g, Carbs: 27g, Protein: 4g

Preparation Time: 10 Minutes

Cooking Time: 27 Minutes

Servings: 4

Ingredents:

1 medium yellow onion, peeled and diced

Water, as needed

2 cloves garlic, peeled and minced

1 tablespoon of ginger, grated

½ jalapeño pepper, deseeded and minced

1 medium head cauliflower, cut into florets

2 medium tomatoes, diced

1-pound (454 g) Yukon Gold potatoes, cut into ½-inch dices

1 teaspoon ground coriander

1 teaspoon ground cumin

1 teaspoon red pepper flakes, crushed

½ teaspoon turmeric

¼ teaspoon ground cloves

2 bay leaves

1 cup green peas

¼ cup chopped cilantro or mint, for garnish

 Directions:

Sauté the onion in a large pot over low to medium heat for 7 to 8 minutes, stirring occasionally. Add water, 1 to 3 tablespoons at a time, to keep it from sticking to the pan.

Stir in the garlic, ginger, and jalapeño pepper and sauté for 3 minutes.

Add the cauliflower, tomatoes, potatoes, coriander, cumin, crushed red pepper flakes, turmeric, cloves, and bay leaves and stir to combine—cover and cook for 12 to 15 minutes, or until the vegetables are soft.

Mix in the peas and cook for an additional 5 minutes.

Remove the bay leaves and sprinkle the chopped cilantro on top for garnish. Serve immediately.

Nutrition: Calories: 175, Fat: 1g, Carbs: 34g, Protein: 6g

5. Kale and Pinto Bean Enchilada Casserole

Preparation Time: 10 Minutes

Cooking Time: 30 Minutes

Servings: 8

Ingredents:

1 teaspoon olive oil (optional)

1 yellow onion, diced

1 bunch kale stemmed and chopped

2 teaspoons of Taco Seasoning

2 to 3 cups cooked pinto beans, or 2 (15-ounce / 425-g) cans pinto beans, drained and rinsed

Sea salt, to taste (optional)

Black pepper, to taste

1 (16-ounce / 454-g) jar salsa (any variety), divided

12 corn tortillas

½ cup cashew queso, or more to taste

Directions:

Preheat the oven to 350°F (205°C). Grease a baking dish with the olive oil, if desired.

Place the onion, kale, taco seasoning, and beans in the dish. Sprinkle with salt (if desired) and pepper. Drizzle half the salsa over the beans. Place the tortillas on top. Scatter with the remaining salsa and cashew queso.

Cover the dish with aluminum foil and bake in the preheated oven for about 30 minutes, or until the vegetables are warm and the salsa bubbles.

Let it cool for 10 minutes before slicing and serving.

Nutrition: Calories: 194 , Fat: 3g, Carbs: 29g, Protein: 10g

6. Potato and Zucchini Casserole

Preparation Time: 10 Minutes

Cooking Time: 1 hour

Servings: 6

Ingredents:

3 large russet potatoes, halved lengthwise and thinly sliced

3 medium zucchinis, halved lengthwise and thinly sliced

¾ cup nutritional yeast

¾ cup diced green or red bell pepper (about one small bell pepper)

¾ cup diced red, white, or yellow onion (about one small onion)

½ cup dry breadcrumbs

¼ cup olive oil (optional)

1½ teaspoons minced garlic (about three small cloves)

Pepper, to taste

Sea salt, to taste (optional)

Directions:

Preheat the oven to 400ºF.

Mix all the ingredients.

Place the mixture in a large cooking pot dish.

Bake in the preheated oven for 1 hour until heated through, stirring once halfway through.

Take off from the oven and allow to cool for 5 minutes before serving.

Nutrition: Calories: 352, Fat: 10g, Carbs: 51g, Protein: 14g

7. Broccoli Casserole with Beans and Walnuts

Preparation Time: 10 Minutes

Cooking Time: 35-40 Minutes

Servings: 4

Ingredents:

¾ cup vegetable broth

2 broccoli heads, crowns, and stalks finely chopped

1 teaspoon of salt (optional)

2 cups cooked pinto or navy beans

1 to 2 tablespoons of brown rice flour or arrowroot flour

1 cup of walnuts, chopped

Directions:

Preheat the oven to 400°F (205°C).

Warm the vegetable broth in a large ovenproof pot over medium heat.

Add the broccoli and season with salt, if desired, then cook for 6 to 8 minutes, stirring occasionally, or until the broccoli is light green.

Add the pinto beans and brown rice flour to the skillet and stir well. Sauté for another 5 to 7 minutes, or until the liquid thickens slightly. Scatter the top with the walnuts.

Transfer the pot to the oven. Bake it until the walnuts are toasted, 20 to 25 minutes.

Let the casserole cool for 8 to 10 minutes in the pot before serving.

Nutrition: Calories: 412, Fat: 20g, Carbs: 43g, Protein: 21g

8. Pistachio Crusted Tofu

Preparation Time: 10 Minutes

Cooking Time: 20 Minutes

Servings: 8

Ingredents:

½ cup roasted, shelled pistachios

¼ cup whole wheat breadcrumbs

1 garlic clove, minced

1 shallot, minced

½ teaspoon of dried tarragon

1 teaspoon of grated lemon zest

Sea salt, to taste (optional)

Black pepper, to taste

1 (16-ounce / 454-g) package sprouted or extra-firm tofu, drained and sliced lengthwise into eight pieces

1 tablespoon of Dijon mustard

1 tablespoon of lemon juice

Directions:

Warm up the oven to 400°F (205°C). Line a baking sheet with parchment paper.

Then place the pistachios in a food processor until they are about the size of the breadcrumbs. Mix the pistachios, breadcrumbs, garlic, shallot, tarragon, and lemon zest in a shallow dish. Sprinkle with salt (if desired) and pepper. Set aside.

Sprinkle the tofu with salt (if desired) and pepper. Mix the mustard and lemon juice in a small bowl and stir well.

Brush all over the tofu with the mustard mixture, then coat each slice with the pistachio mixture.

Arrange the tofu on the baking sheet. Scatter any remaining pistachio mixture over the slices.

Bake in the warmed oven for about 18 to 20 minutes, or until the tofu is browned and crispy.

Serve hot.

Nutrition: Calories: 159, Fat: 9g, Carbs: 8g, Protein: 10g

9. Strawberry Chocolate Shake

Preparation Time: 10 Minutes

Cooking Time: 0 Minutes

Servings: 1

Ingredients:

1 cup water

1 cup frozen strawberries

1 oz baby arugula

½ avocado

½ teaspoon of vanilla extract

1 tablespoon of cacao powder

Directions

In a food processor, add in all the ingredients and blitz until smooth and creamy. Add ice for a thicker consistency, if desired. Serve immediately!

Nutrition: Calories 233, Fat: 7g, Carbs: 41g, Protein: 2g

10. Power Green Smoothie

Preparation Time: 10 minutes

Cooking Time: 0 minutes

Servings: 2

Ingredients:

1 little gem lettuce, roughly chopped

2 cups almond milk

1 cup baby spinach, chopped

2 Medjool dates, pitted

A few ice cubes (optional)

Directions:

In a blender, mix in all the ingredients and pulse until completely smooth. Pour into two glasses and serve immediately.

Nutrition: Calories 114, Fat: 4g, Carbs: 23g, Protein: 2g

Preparation Time: 10 minutes

Cooking Time: 0 minutes

Servings: 1

Ingredients:

1 cup water

1 green apple, cored and chopped

1 Medjool date, pitted

1 tablespoon of cacao powder

½ tablespoon of cinnamon powder

2 tablespoons of pea protein powder

4-5 ice cubes

Directions:

In a blender, mix water, apples, date, cacao powder, cinnamon, and protein powder. Blitz until completely smooth.

Add in the ice and pulse again until a thick and smooth texture is obtained. Serve right away!

Nutrition: Calories 253, Fat: 3g, Carbs: 49g, Protein: 15g

12. Morning Matcha Smoothie

Preparation Time: 10 minutes

Cooking Time: 0 minutes

Servings: 1

Ingredients:

1 cup almond milk

1 kiwi

½ avocado

½ inch fresh ginger, peeled (optional; add to taste)

1 handful of fresh baby spinach

½ teaspoon matcha powder

Directions:

In a blender, mix all ingredients and blitz until smooth. Add some pitted dates for more sweetness, if desired. Serve immediately!

Nutrition: Calories 316, Fat: 10g, Carbs: 61g, Protein: 8g

13. Ginger & Apple Green Smoothie

Preparation Time: 5 minutes

Cooking Time: 0 minutes

Servings: 2

Ingredients:

1 cup of cucumber, chopped

1 cup curly endive

1 apple, peeled and cored

2 tablespoons of lime juice

1 cups soy milk

½-inch piece peeled fresh ginger

1 tablespoon of chia seeds

1 cup unsweetened coconut yogurt

Directions:

Put in a food processor the cucumber, curly endive, apple, lime juice, soy milk, ginger, chia seeds, and coconut yogurt. Blend until smooth. Serve.

Nutrition: Calories 165, Fat: 4g, Carbs: 28g, Protein: 7g

14. Grilled Cauliflower Steaks

Preparation Time: 10 Minutes

Cooking Time: 57 Minutes

Servings: 4

Ingredents:

2 medium heads cauliflower

2 medium shallots, peeled and minced

Water, as needed

1 clove garlic, peeled and minced

½ teaspoon ground fennel

½ teaspoon minced sage

½ teaspoon crushed red pepper flakes

½ cup green lentils, rinsed

2 cups of low-sodium vegetable broth

Salt, to taste (optional)

Freshly ground black pepper, to taste

Chopped parsley, for garnish

Directions:

On a flat work surface, cut each of the cauliflower heads in half through the stem, then trim each half, so you get a 1-inch-thick steak.

Arrange each piece on a baking sheet and set aside. You can reserve the extra cauliflower florets for other uses.

Sauté the shallots in a medium saucepan over medium heat for 10 minutes, stirring occasionally. Add water, 1 to 3 tablespoons at a time, to keep the shallots from sticking.

Stir in the garlic, fennel, sage, red pepper flakes, and lentils and cook for 3 minutes.

Pour into the vegetable broth and bring to a boil over high heat.

Grill the cauliflower steaks for about 7 minutes per side until evenly browned.

Transfer the cauliflower steaks to a plate and spoon the purée over them. Serve garnished with the parsley.

Nutrition: Calories: 105, Fat: 1g, Carbs: 18g, Protein: 5g

15. Treacle Buckwheat Granola

Preparation Time: 15 minutes

Cooking Time: 0 minutes

Servings: 1

Ingredients:

1 cup buckwheat groats

½ cup chopped pecans

½ cup shredded coconut

1 tablespoon of chia seeds

1 tablespoon of date sugar

A pinch of sea salt

½ teaspoon of ground cardamon

½ cup olive oil

½ cup black treacle (or molasses)

Directions:

Preheat oven to 320 F. In a bowl, add the all the ingredients and stir to combine.

In a small saucepan over medium-low heat, warm the oil and black treacle until melted and well combined. Spread the mixture evenly onto a lined baking sheet and bake for 25-30 minutes, stirring halfway through for an even baking.

Nutrition: Calories 270, Fat: 8g, Carbs: 52g, Protein: 9g

16. Cinnamon Buckwheat with Walnuts

Preparation Time: 10 minutes

Cooking Time: 20 minutes

Servings: 1

Ingredients:

1 cup of almond milk

1 cup of water

1 cup of buckwheat groats, rinsed

1 teaspoon of cinnamon

¼ cup of walnuts, chopped

2 tablespoon of pure date syrup

Directions:

Place almond milk, water, and buckwheat in a pot over medium heat. Lower the heat and simmer covered for 15 minutes. Allow sitting covered for 5 minutes. Mix in the cinnamon, walnuts, and date syrup. Serve warm.

Nutrition: Calories 245, Fat: 9g, Carbs: 37g, Protein: 7g

17. Instant Savory Gigante Beans

Preparation Time: 10-30 Minutes

Cooking Time: 55 Minutes

Servings: 6

Ingredents:

1 lb. Gigante Beans, soaked overnight

½ cup of olive oil

1 onion, sliced

2 cloves garlic, crushed or minced

1 red bell pepper, cut into ⅓ inch pieces

2 carrots, sliced

½ teaspoon of salt and ground black pepper

2 tomatoes peeled, grated

1 tablespoon of celery, chopped

1 tablespoon of tomato paste (or ketchup)

¾ teaspoon of sweet paprika

1 teaspoon of oregano

1 cup vegetable broth

Directions:

Soak Gigante beans overnight.

Press the SAUTÉ button on your Instant Pot and heat the oil.

Sauté onion, garlic, sweet pepper, carrots with a pinch of salt for 3 - 4 minutes; stir occasionally.

Add rinsed Gigante beans into your Instant Pot along with all remaining ingredients and stir well.

Latch lid into place and set on the MANUAL setting for 25 minutes.

When the beep sounds, quick release the pressure by pressing Cancel and twisting the steam handle to the Venting position.

Taste and adjust seasonings to taste.

Serve warm or cold.

Keep refrigerated.

Nutrition: Calories 502, Fat: 6g, Carbs: 31g, Protein: 9g

18. Instant Turmeric Risotto

Preparation Time: 10-30 Minutes

Cooking Time: 40 Minutes

Servings: 4

Ingredents:

4 tablespoons of olive oil

1 cup of onion

1 teaspoon of minced garlic

2 cups of long-grain rice

3 cups of vegetable broth

½ teaspoon of paprika (smoked)

½ teaspoon of turmeric

½ teaspoon of nutmeg

2 Tablespoon of fresh basil leaves chopped

Salt and ground black pepper to taste

Directions:

Press the SAUTÉ button on your Instant Pot and heat oil.

Sauté the onion and garlic with a pinch of salt until softened.

Add the rice and all leftover ingredients and stir well.

Lock the lid into place and set on and select the RICE button for 10 minutes.

Press Cancel when the timer beeps and carefully flip the Quick Release valve to let the pressure out.

Taste and adjust seasonings to taste.

Serve.

Nutrition: Calories 559, Fat: 6g, Carbs: 29g, Protein: 9g

19. Nettle Soup with Rice

Preparation Time: 10-30 Minutes

Cooking Time: 40 Minutes

Servings: 5

Ingredients:

3 tablespoons of of olive oil

2 onions, finely chopped

2 cloves garlic, finely chopped

Salt and freshly ground black pepper

4 medium potatoes, cut into cubes

1 cup of rice

1 tablespoon of arrowroot

2 cups of vegetable broth

2 cups of water

1 bunch of young nettle leaves packed

½ cup fresh parsley, finely chopped

1 teaspoon of cumin

Directions:

Heat olive oil in a large pot.

Sauté onion and garlic with a pinch of salt until softened.

Add potato, rice, and arrowroot; sauté for 2 to 3 minutes.

Pour broth and water, stir well, cover and cook over medium heat for about 20 minutes.

Cook for about 30 to 45 minutes.

Add young nettle leaves, parsley, and cumin; stir and cook for 5 to 7 minutes.

Move the soup in a blender and blend until combined well.

Taste and adjust salt and pepper.

Serve hot.

Nutrition: Calories 421, Fat: 8g, Carbs: 18g, Protein: 10g

20. Okra with Grated Tomatoes

Preparation Time: 10-30 Minutes

Cooking Time: 3 Hours and 10 Minutes

Servings: 4

Ingredents:

2 lbs. fresh okra, cleaned

2 onions, finely chopped

2 cloves garlic, finely sliced

2 carrots, sliced

2 ripe tomatoes, grated

1 cup of water

4 tablespoon of olive oil

Salt and ground black pepper

1 tablespoon of fresh parsley, finely chopped

Directions:

Add okra in your Crock-Pot: sprinkle with a pinch of salt and pepper. Add in chopped onion, garlic, carrots, and grated tomatoes; stir well. Pour water and oil, season with the salt, pepper, and give a good stir.

Covering and cook on LOW for 2-4 hours or until tender.

Open the lid and add fresh parsley; stir. Taste and adjust salt and pepper.

Serve hot.

 Nutrition: Calories 249, Fat: 8g, Carbs: 21g, Protein: 8g

21. Oven-Baked Smoked Lentil Burgers

Preparation Time: 10-30 Minutes

Cooking Time: 1 Hour and 20 Minutes

Servings: 6

 Ingredents:

1 ½ cups of dried lentils

3 cups of water

Salt and ground black pepper to taste

2 tablespoons of olive oil

1 onion, finely diced

2 cloves of garlic, minced

1 cup of button mushrooms sliced

2 tablespoons of tomato paste

½ teaspoon of fresh basil, finely chopped

1 cup of chopped almonds

3 teaspoon of balsamic vinegar

3 tablespoon of coconut amino

1 teaspoon of liquid smoke

¾ cup silken tofu soft

¾ cup corn starch

Directions:

Cook lentils in salted water until tender or for about 30-35 minutes; rinse, drain, and set aside.

Heat oil in a frying skillet and sauté onion, garlic, and mushrooms for 4 to 5 minutes; stir occasionally.

Stir in the tomato paste, salt, basil, salt, and black pepper; cook for 2 to 3 minutes.

Stir in almonds, vinegar, coconut amino, liquid smoke, and lentils.

Remove from heat and stir in blended tofu and corn starch.

Keep stirring until all ingredients combined well.

Form mixture into patties and refrigerate for an hour.

Preheat oven to 350 F.

Line a baking dish with parchment paper and arrange patties on the pan.

Bake for 20 to 25 minutes.

Serve hot with buns, green salad, tomato sauce, etc.

Nutrition: Calories 532, Fat: 7g, Carbs: 20g, Protein: 6g

22. Powerful Spinach and Mustard Leaves Puree

Preparation Time: 10-30 Minutes

Cooking Time: 50 Minutes

Servings: 4

Ingredents:

2 Tablespoon of almond butter

One onion finely diced

2 Tablespoon of minced garlic

1 teaspoon of salt and black pepper (or to taste)

1 lb. mustard leaves cleaned rinsed

1 lb. frozen spinach thawed

1 teaspoon of coriander

1 teaspoon of ground cumin

½ cup almond milk

Directions:

Press the SAUTÉ button on your Instant Pot and heat the almond butter. Sauté onion, garlic, and a pinch of salt for 2-3 minutes; stir occasionally.

Add spinach and the mustard greens and stir for a minute or two. Season with the salt and pepper, coriander, and cumin; give a good stir.

Lock lid into place and set on the MANUAL setting for 15 minutes.

Use Quick Release - turn the valve from sealing to venting to release the pressure.

Move mixture to a blender, add almond milk and blend until smooth.

Taste and adjust seasonings. Serve.

Nutrition: Calories 290, Fat: 6g, Carbs: 26g, Protein: 9g

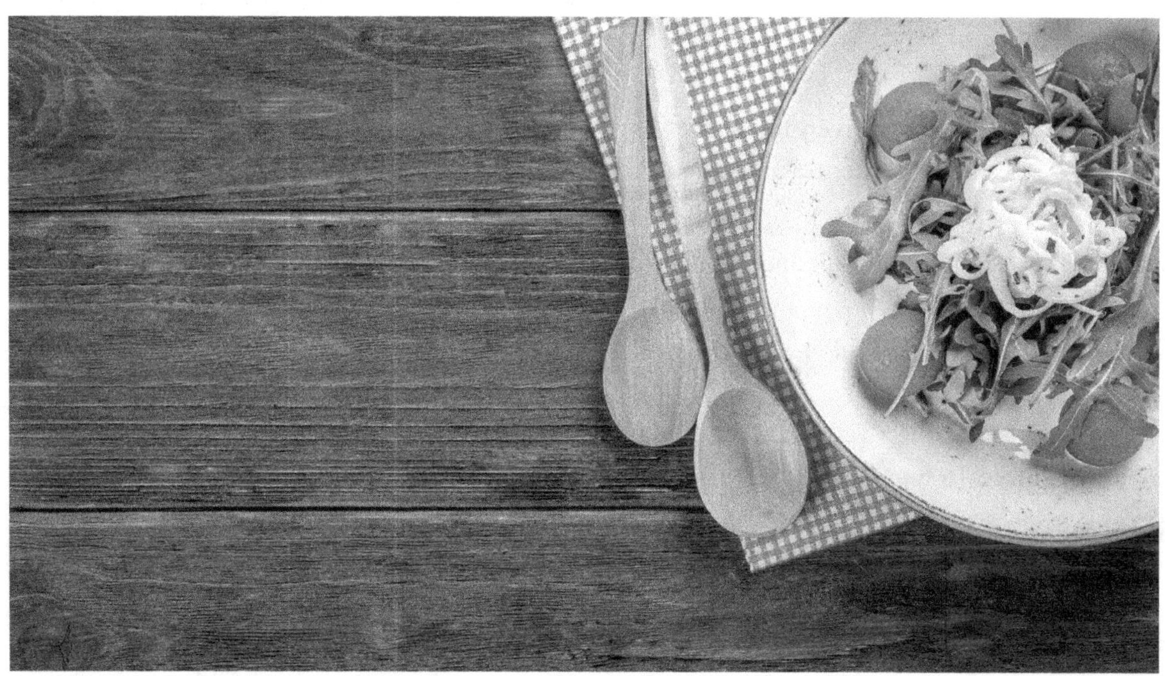

23. Roasted Chickpeas

Preparation Time: 10 minutes

Cooking Time: 9 hours 20 minutes

Servings: 12

Ingredients:

1 lb. dried chickpeas (garbanzo beans)

2 tablespoons of. Olive oil

Kosher salt, to taste

Directions:

In a big container, put the chickpeas and pour a couple inches of cold water to cover, then allow it to stand for 8 hours to overnight.

Let the chickpeas drain and pat it dry.

Set an oven to preheat to 200°C (400°F).

In a bowl, toss together the salt, olive oil and chickpeas until coated evenly, then spread it on a baking tray in a single layer.

Let it roast in the preheated oven for about 40 minutes, mixing every 8 minutes, until the chickpeas become crisp and turns brown.

Toss the chickpeas with more salt and allow it to fully cool.

Nutrition: Calories 509, Fat: 2g, Carbs: 48g, Protein: 1g

24. Mango Salsa

Preparation Time: 15 minutes
Cooking Time: 1hour 15 minutes

Servings: 6

Ingredients:

4 mangos, peeled, seeded, and diced

1 (15 oz.) can black beans, rinsed and drained

1 (10 oz.) can white shoepeg corn, drained

2 tablespoon ofs. Chopped fresh cilantro

1 lime, juiced

Salt and pepper to taste

Directions:

Mix pepper, salt, lime juice, cilantro, corn, black beans and diced mango in a bowl.

Chill for at least 1 hour; serve.

Nutrition: Calories 210, Fat: 2g, Carbs: 18g, Protein: 6g

Preparation Time: 15 minutes

Cooking Time: 15 minutes

Servings: 4

Ingredients:

20 green grapes

1 tablespoon of. cream cheese, softened

10 miniature semisweet chocolate chips

Skewers

Directions:

Choose 5 nicest looking grapes.

Put on each one with 2 small dollops of cream cheese to make eyes and stick in mini chocolate chips for the pupils.

Thread 3-4 grapes lengthways onto a skewer, depending on the length of your skewers, followed by the grape with the eyes horizontally.

Repeat with other grapes.

Nutrition: Calories 159, Fat: 2g, Carbs: 32g, Protein: 4g

Preparation Time: 20 minutes

Cooking Time: 20 minutes

Servings: 16

Ingredients:

8 hard-boiled large eggs

3 tbsps. Fat-free mayonnaise

2 tbsps. Lemon juice

4 tsps. Minced fresh tarragon

1 tbsp. chopped green onion

1/4 tsp. salt

1/4 tsp. hot pepper sauce

⅛ tsp. cayenne pepper

1 can (6 oz.) crabmeat, drained, flaked and cartilage removed

Directions:

Halve the eggs lengthwise.

Take out the yolks, then put aside the 4 yolks and egg whites

Mash the reserved yolks in a big bowl. Stir in cayenne, hot pepper sauce, salt, onion, tarragon, lemon juice and mayonnaise.

Mix in crab until well blended. Pipe or stuff it into egg whites, then chill it in the fridge until ready to serve.

Nutrition: Calories 321, Fat: 1g, Carbs: 23g, Protein: 5g

27. Cinnamon Toasties

Preparation Time: 10 minutes

Cooking Time: 20 minutes

Servings: 4

Ingredients:

8 slices bread

¼ cup reduced-fat cream cheese

Refrigerated butter-flavored spray

3 tablespoon ofs. Sugar

1-½ teaspoon ofs. Ground cinnamon

Directions:

Use a rolling pin to flatten bread.

Spread half of the slices with cream cheese on one side; put remaining bread on top.

Slice into four squares each. Spritz butter-flavored spray on both sides.

Mix cinnamon and sugar in a small bowl; include bread squares and flip to cover both sides.

Put on an ungreased baking sheet. Bake for 8-10 minutes at 350° or until golden and puffed. Serve right away.

Nutrition: Calories 231, Fat: 1g, Carbs: 42g, Protein: 1g

28. Fusion Peach Salsa

Preparation Time: 5 minutes

Cooking Time: 5 minutes

Servings: 4

Ingredients:

2 (15 oz.) cans peaches, drained and chopped

2 green onions with tops, thinly sliced

2 teaspoon ofs. Chopped fresh cilantro

2 tablespoon ofs. Lime juice

¼ teaspoon of. Asian five-spice powder

2 teaspoon ofs. Garlic chile paste

⅛ teaspoon of. white pepper

Directions:

Mix together lime juice, cilantro, green onion and peaches in a medium bowl, then combine in white pepper, garlic Chile paste and five-spice powder.

Chill with a cover until serving.

Nutrition: Calories 108, Fat: 2g, Carbs: 39g, Protein: 2g

29. Basil and Pesto Hummus

Preparation Time: 10 minutes

Cooking Time: 10 minutes

Servings: 5

Ingredients:

1 (16 oz.) garbanzo beans (chickpeas), drained and rinsed

½ cup basil leaves

1 clove garlic

1 tablespoon of. olive oil

½ teaspoon of. balsamic vinegar

½ teaspoon of. soy sauce

Salt and ground black pepper to taste

Directions:

In a food processor, mix garlic, basil, and garbanzo beans, then pulse a few times.

Scrape down the sides of the processor bowl using a spatula. Pulse again while drizzling in the olive oil.

Stir in soy sauce and vinegar, and process until incorporated.

Sprinkle pepper and salt to season.

Nutrition: Calories 120, Fat: 1g, Carbs: 12g, Protein: 1g

30. Sweet Potato Chips

Preparation Time: 5 minutes

Cooking Time: 15 minutes

Servings: 2

Ingredients:

1 sweet potato, thinly sliced

2 teaspoon ofs. Olive oil, or as needed

Coarse sea salt

Directions:

Mix olive oil and sweet potato slices in a big bowl and coat by tossing.

Place the sweet potato slices in one layer on a big plate that's microwave safe. Season using salt.

Cook until slightly browned, crisp, and dry in a microwave for 5 minutes.

Cool the chips on a plate then transfer to a bowl. Repeat steps with leftover sweet potato slices.

Nutrition: Calories 149, Fat: 1g, Carbs: 20g, Protein: 3g

31. Mango Apple Mania Salsa

Preparation Time: 30 minutes

Cooking Time: 40 minutes

Servings: 24

Ingredients:

1 red onion, peeled and halved

12 mangos - peeled, seeded, and diced

½ head garlic, pressed

1 Apple

3 habanero peppers, seeded and minced

1 bunch fresh cilantro, chopped

2 tablespoon ofs. Apple cider vinegar

Salt to taste

Directions:

Preheat outdoor grill to high heat.

Oil the grate lightly. Put onion onto grill.

Cook until blackened slightly.

Dice onion. In a mixing bowl, mix apple cider, cilantro, habanero, garlic, Apple and mango. Season with salt to taste.

Nutrition: Calories 129, Fat: 2g, Carbs: 33g, Protein: 3g

32. Marinated Mushrooms

Preparation Time: 15 minutes

Cooking Time: 25 minutes

Servings: 8

Ingredients:

1 cup red wine

½ cup red wine vinegar

⅓ cup olive oil

2 tablespoon ofs. Brown sugar

2 cloves garlic, minced

1 teaspoon of. crushed red pepper flakes

¼ cup red bell pepper, diced

1 lb. small fresh mushrooms, washed and trimmed

¼ cup chopped green onions

¼ teaspoon of. dried oregano

½ teaspoon of. salt

¼ teaspoon of. ground black pepper

Directions:

Mix together the mushrooms, red pepper flakes, bell pepper, garlic, sugar, oil, vinegar and wine in a saucepan on medium heat, then boil.

Put cover and put aside to let it cool.

Mix in pepper, salt, oregano and green onions once cooled. Serve it at room temperature or chilled.

Nutrition: Calories 212, Fat: 3g, Carbs: 18g, Protein: 4g

33. Layered Creamy Taco Dip

Preparation Time: 20 minutes

Cooking Time: 20 minutes

Servings: 4

Ingredients:

1 package (8 oz.) fat-free cream cheese

½ cup reduced-fat sour cream

¼ cup fat-free mayonnaise

2 teaspoon ofs. Taco seasoning

1 cup taco sauce

2 cups shredded part-skim mozzarella cheese

1 medium green pepper, diced

3 green onions, chopped

1 medium tomato, diced

Tortilla chips

Directions:

Beat taco seasoning, mayonnaise, sour cream and cream cheese in a bowl till smooth. Transfer into a 12-inch round serving plate and spread.

Top off with taco sauce and spread. Sprinkle with tomato, onions, green pepper and mozzarella cheese.

Store in the fridge, covered, till serving. Serve with tortilla chips.

Nutrition: Calories 223, Fat: 6g, Carbs: 17g, Protein: 2g

34. Garlic Spinach Balls

Preparation Time: 25 minutes

Cooking Time: 40 minutes

Servings: 8

Ingredients:

2 cups crushed seasoned stuffing

1 cup finely chopped onion

4 large eggs, lightly beaten

¾ cup butter, melted

½ cup grated Parmesan cheese

1 garlic clove, minced

1-½ teaspoon ofs. dried thyme

¼ teaspoon of. salt

¼ teaspoon of. pepper

2 packages (10 oz. each) frozen chopped spinach, thawed and squeezed dry

Directions:

Mix together the initial 9 ingredients in a big bowl.

Mix in spinach until combined. Roll it into 1-inch balls, then put it in a greased 15x10x1-inch baking pan.

Let it bake for 15-20 minutes at 350 degrees or until it turns golden brown in color.

Nutrition: Calories 244, Fat: 2g, Carbs: 29g, Protein: 2g

35. Apple Salsa

Preparation Time: 20 minutes

Cooking Time: 1 hour 20 minutes

Servings: 40

Ingredients:

Tomatoes

Apple

Onion

Sugar

Cilantro

Vinegar

½ teaspoon of. salt

½ teaspoon of. black pepper

2 cloves garlic, minced

Directions:

In a bowl, stir together garlic, pepper, salt, cider vinegar, lime juice, cilantro, sugar, onion, apple and tomatoes, then chill about 1 hour before serving.

Nutrition: Calories 251, Fat: 9g, Carbs: 12g, Protein: 6g

36. Stuffed Dates

Preparation Time: 15 minutes

Cooking Time: 15 minutes

Servings: 10

Ingredients:

3 oz. reduced-fat cream cheese

¼ cup confectioners' sugar

2 teaspoon ofs. grated orange zest

30 pitted dates

Directions:

Beat the orange zest, confectioner's sugar and cream cheese in a small bowl until combined.

Make a slit in the middle of each date carefully, then fill it with the cream cheese mixture. Put cover and let it chill in the fridge for a minimum of 1 hour prior to serving.

Nutrition: Calories 200, Fat: 7g, Carbs: 6g, Protein: 5g

Preparation Time: 20 minutes

Cooking Time: 25 minutes

Servings: 10

Ingredients:

3 packages (6 oz. each) fresh baby spinach, chopped

1 teaspoon of. water

½ cup crumbled feta cheese

1 plum tomatoes, seeded and chopped

¼ cup finely chopped red onion

3 tablespoon ofs. fat-free mayonnaise

3 tablespoon ofs. fat-free sour cream

1 garlic clove, minced

½ teaspoon of. salt

½ teaspoon of. dill weed

20 slices French baguette (½ inch thick)

Directions:

Mix spinach with water in a big microwave-safe bowl. Cover and microwave at high heat until spinach is diminished, for 1 ½ to 2 minutes, stir twice then drain and squeeze.

Mix in the dill weed, salt, garlic, sour cream, mayonnaise, onion, tomato, and feta cheese; put aside.

Lay bread on a baking tray. Put the tray 4 inches away from the heat source and broil until bread is toasted slightly, for 1 to 2 minutes. Add about 1 tablespoon of. of the spinach mixture over each bread. Broil for 3 to 4 more minutes until cooked through.

Nutrition: Calories 159, Fat: 11g, Carbs: 11g, Protein: 3g

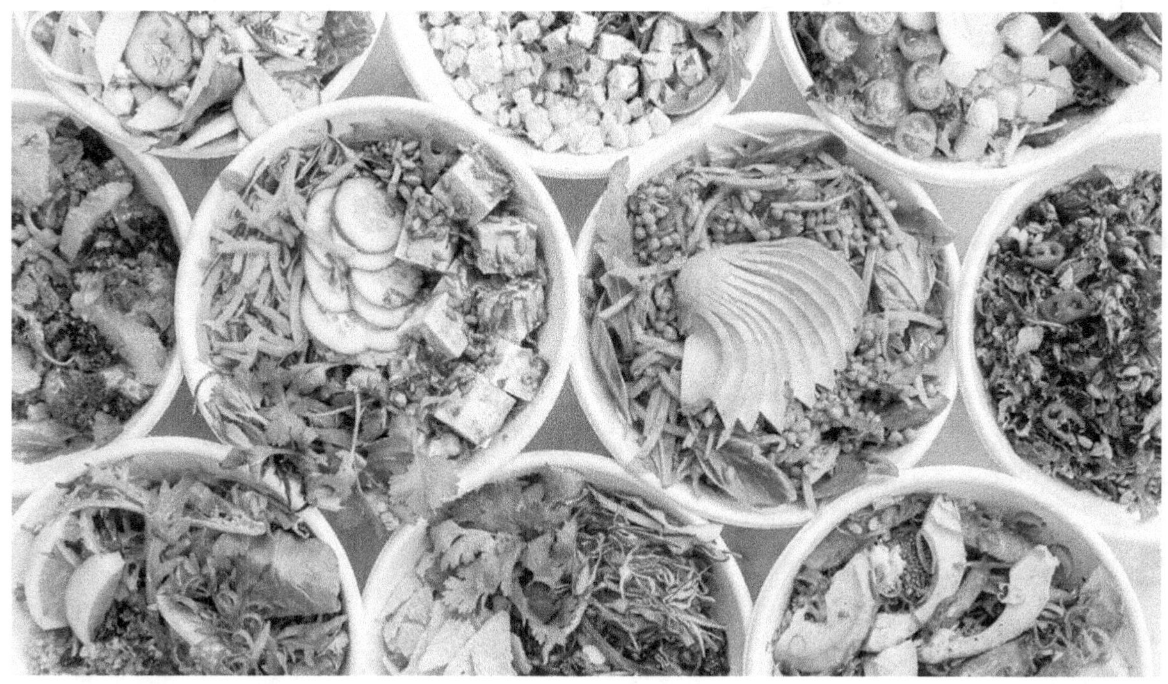

38. Mediterranean fish and quinoa soup

Preparation time: 5 minutes

Cooking time: 40 minutes

Servings: 3

Ingredients:

1lb cod fillets, cubed

1 onion, chopped

3 tomatoes, chopped

½ cup quinoa, rinsed

1 red pepper, chopped

1 carrot, chopped

½ cup black olives, pitted and sliced

1 garlic clove, crushed

3 tablespoon of extra virgin olive oil

A pinch of cayenne pepper

1 bay leaf

1 teaspoon of dried thyme

1 teaspoon of dried dill

½ teaspoon of pepper

½ cup white wine

4 cups water

Salt and black pepper, to taste

½ cup fresh parsley, finely cut

Directions:

Heat the olive oil over medium heat and sauté the onion, red pepper, garlic and carrot until tender.

Stir in the cayenne pepper, bay leaf, herbs, salt and pepper.

Add the white wine, water, quinoa and tomatoes and bring to a boil.

Reduce heat, cover, and cook for 10 minutes.

Stir in olives and the fish and cook for another 10 minutes.

Stir in parsley and serve hot.

Nutrition: Calories 324, Fat: 6g, Carbs: 19g, Protein: 6g

39. Bean stew

Preparation time: 5 minutes

Cooking time: 35 minutes

Servings: 3

Ingredients:

50g of kale, chopped roughly

½ bird's eye chilli, chopped finely (optional)

40g of buckwheat

50g of red onion, chopped finely

1 garlic clove, chopped finely

1 tablespoon of of roughly chopped parsley

200ml vegetable stock

1 teaspoon of of herbes de provence

200g of tinned mixed beans

1 teaspoon of of tomato purée

1 x 400g tin of chopped Italian tomatoes

30g celery, trimmed and chopped finely

1 tablespoon of of extra virgin olive oil

30g of carrot, peeled and chopped finely

Directions:

Heat the oil in a medium sized saucepan placed over medium low heat.

Add in the onion, celery, chilli, carrot, garlic and herbs (if using) until the onions are soft enough but not coloured.

Add the stock, tomato purée, and tomatoes and bring to a boil. Put in the beans and allow for 30 minutes simmering. Add the kales and cook for 5-10 minutes or until the kale is tender, and then add in parsley.

As it cools, cook the buckwheat as per the directions on the packet.

Drain the buckwheat and serve with the cooked stew.

Nutrition: Calories 324, Fat: 4g, Carbs: 17g, Protein: 4g

40. Pork with pak choi

Preparation time: 5 minutes

Cooking time: 40 minutes

Servings: 3

Ingredients:

100g of shiitake mushrooms, sliced

1 tablespoon of of corn flour

200g pak choi or choi sum-cut into thin slices

125ml of chicken stock

1 tablespoon of tomato purée

1 teaspoon of brown sugar

1 clove garlic, peeled and crushed

1 shallot, peeled and sliced

100g of bean sprouts

1 tablespoon of of water

400g of pork mince (10% fat)

1 thumb (5cm) fresh ginger -peeled and grated

400g of firm tofu, cut into large cubes

1 tablespoon of rice wine

1 tablespoon of soy sauce

A large handful (20g) of parsley, chopped

1 tablespoon of rapeseed oil

Directions:

Place the tofu on kitchen paper, cover it with kitchen paper, and then set it aside.

In a small bowl, mix water and corn flour and remove the lumps.

Add in rice wine, brown sugar, chicken stock, tomato puree, and soy sauce.

Also, add in the crushed ginger and garlic them mix.

Place a large frying pan or wok on high heat and add oil to it.

Add the mushrooms and stir-fry for 2 to 3 minutes until cooked and glossy.

Using a slotted spoon, remove the mushrooms from the pan and let them rest.

Add tofu to the pan, fry it until it is brown on all sides, remove it with a slotted spoon when done and set aside.

Add the pak choi to your pan or wok, and stir-fry for about 2 minutes and, then add the mince.

Cook it until it cooks through and then add the sauce.

Reduce the heat a notch and allow the sauce to bubble around the meat for 1-2 minutes.

Add the tofu, beansprouts, and mushrooms to the pan and warm them all through.

Remove it from the heat and mix in parsley then serve right away.

Nutrition: Calories 178, Fat: 4g, Carbs: 19g, Protein: 5g

41. Chicken soup

Preparation time: 5 minutes

Cooking time: 30 minutes

Servings: 3

Ingredients:

1 teaspoon of of smoked paprika

300ml passata

Salt and freshly ground black pepper

1 teaspoon of dried mixed herbs

1 400g can of black beans, drained

2 cloves garlic, peeled and crushed

1 carrot, peeled and roughly chopped

1 litre of water

1 teaspoon of mild chilli powder

1 red chilli, deseeded then finely chopped

½ teaspoon of of turmeric

30g (large handful) of flat leaf parsley, chopped

1 x 400g can chopped tomatoes

1 teaspoon of of paprika

½ teaspoon of of ground cumin

1 green pepper, deseeded and chopped

1 x 400g can kidney beans, drained

4 chicken drumsticks

2 shallots, peeled then roughly chopped

Directions:

Take a large saucepan and add in the chicken drumsticks, carrot, and shallots.

Pour in the water and let it simmer.

Allow to cook for 20 minutes, and then remove the chicken drumsticks with a spoon (slotted) and set it aside to cool.

Add in the chopped tomatoes, garlic, passata, chilli, and green pepper, and let it simmer again.

Put in the dried herbs, paprika, turmeric, smoked paprika, chilli powder, and cumin, then simmer again for 30 minutes.

Pull off the skin from the chicken then pinch as much chicken as possible from the bone.

Shred the chicken meat, place it on the pan along with the kidney beans and black beans, and cook for five minutes.

Remove from the heat, add parsley, and stir it in.

Season with pepper and salt (to taste).

Nutrition: Calories 389, Fat: 5g, Carbs: 14g, Protein: 2g

42. Beef with red wine and herb-roasted potatoes

Preparation time: 5 minutes

Cooking time: 60 minutes

Servings: 3

Ingredients:

40ml of red wine

1 tablespoon of of extra virgin olive oil

1 clove of garlic, finely chopped

5g of parsley, finely chopped

50g of red onions-sliced to rings

50g of sliced kale

1 teaspoon of of corn flour dissolved in 1 tablespoon of of water

100g of potatoes, peeled then cut into 2cm chunks

150ml of beef stock

1 teaspoon of of tomato purée

150g of beefsteak

Directions:

Preheat your oven to 220 degrees.

Boil the potatoes for 5 minutes then drain.

Place them in a roasting tin together with a teaspoon of of oil and let them roast for 35 to 45 minutes.

Make sure to turn them every ten minutes.

Once done, take them out and mix them with parsley.

Over medium heat, fry the onion in a teaspoon of of oil for 5 to 7 minutes.

Steam the kale for 2 to 3 minutes then drain.

Fry the garlic in a teaspoon of of oil for a minute, add the kale, and stir-fry for 1 to 2 more minutes.

Smear the beef with ½ teaspoon of of oil and fry it in a hot pan over medium heat until cooked as desired.

Remove it and set aside.

Pour wine onto the hot pan and reduce the heat to simmer the wine until syrupy.

Add tomato purée and stock, let it boil, and add the corn flour paste to thicken.

Serve the beef with onion rings, roast potatoes, red wine sauce, kale, and enjoy.

Nutrition: Calories 211, Fat: 6g, Carbs: 12g, Protein: 9g

43. Salmon salad with mint dressing

Preparation time: 5 minutes

Cooking time: 30 minutes

Servings: 3

Ingredients:

1 small handful (10g) of parsley, chopped roughly

2 radishes, trimmed and thinly sliced

40g of young spinach leaves

5cm piece (50g) cucumber, cut into chunks

40g of mixed salad leaves

2 spring onions, trimmed then sliced

1 salmon fillet (130g)

For the dressing:

1 tablespoon of of rice vinegar

1 teaspoon of of low-fat mayonnaise

Salt and freshly ground black pepper, to taste 2mint leaves, finely chopped

1 tablespoon of of natural yoghurt

Directions:

Preheat your oven to 200 degrees. Place salmon fillets on a baking tray and allow them to bake for about 16-18 minutes.

Remove from the oven and then let them rest (salmon is ok served hot or cold when added to the salad).

Remove the skin of your salmon (if it has one) after cooking.

Mix the mayonnaise, mint leaves, rice wine vinegar, salt, yoghurt, and pepper in a small bowl and let it stand for 5 minutes to let the flavour deepen.

Place the salad leaves with the spinach on top of a plate and top with the radishes, spring onions, cucumber, and parsley.

Flake the salmon onto the salad then drizzle the dressing over.

Nutrition: Calories 245, Fat: 2g, Carbs: 10g, Protein: 3g

44. Hearty quinoa and spinach breakfast casserole

Preparation time: 5 minutes

Cooking time: 20 minutes

Servings: 3

Ingredients:

1 cup cooked quinoa

3-4 spring onions, finely chopped

5 oz frozen chopped spinach, thawed and squeezed dry

½ zucchini, peeled and shredded

5 eggs

½ cup milk

4 tablespoon of extra virgin olive oil

salt and black pepper, to taste

1 cup cheddar cheese, grated

Directions:

In a large bowl combine eggs, milk, salt and pepper.

In a deep casserole dish heat the olive oil.

Cook the onions, zucchini and spinach, stirring constantly, until lightly cooked.

Add in the quinoa and combine everything well.

Pour the egg mixture over and then top with cheddar cheese.

Bake in a preheated to 350 f oven for 20 minutes.

Nutrition: Calories 211, Fat: 2g, Carbs: 10g, Protein: 2g

45. Quick quinoa vegetable scramble

Preparation time: 5 minutes

Cooking time: 30 minutes

Servings: 3

Ingredients:

½ cup cooked quinoa

½ small onion, chopped

2 tomatoes, diced

1 large red pepper, chopped

5 eggs

½ cup crumbled feta

4 tablespoon of extra virgin olive oil

Black pepper, to taste

Salt, to taste

Directions:

In a large pan, sauté onion over medium heat for 1-2 minutes, stirring.

Add in tomatoes and red pepper and cook until the mixture is almost dry.

Stir in quinoa, feta and eggs and cook until well mixed and not too liquid.

Season with black pepper and serve.

Nutrition: Calories 234, Fat: 2g, Carbs: 19g, Protein: 3g

46. Coconut and quinoa banana pudding

Preparation time: 5 minutes

Cooking time: 30 minutes

Servings: 3

Ingredients:

1 cup quinoa

3 cups coconut milk

3 ripe bananas

¼ cup flaked unsweetened coconut

4 tablespoon of sugar

1 teaspoon of vanilla extract

Directions:

Wash and cook quinoa according to package directions.

When ready remove from heat and set aside.

In a separate bowl blend sugar, milk and bananas until smooth.

Add to the quinoa.

Heat over medium heat, string, until creamy.

Stir in vanilla and coconut flakes and serve warm.

Nutrition: Calories 211, Fat: 3g, Carbs: 12g, Protein: 9g

47. Chicken with kale and chilli salsa

Preparation time: 5 minutes

Cooking time: 40 minutes

Servings: 3

Ingredients:

50g of buckwheat

1 teaspoon of of chopped fresh ginger

Juice of ½ lemon, divided

Turmeric

Kale

Onion

Olive oil

Tomato

Parsley

Chilli

Directions:

Start with the salsa: remove the eye out of the tomato and finely chop it, making sure to keep as much of the liquid as you can.

Mix it with the chilli, parsley, and lemon juice.

You could add everything to a blender for different results.

Heat your oven to 220F.

Marinate the chicken with a little oil, 1 teaspoon of of turmeric, and the lemon juice.

Let it rest for 5-10 minutes.

Heat a pan over medium heat until it is hot then add marinated chicken and allow it to cook for a minute on both sides until it is pale gold).

Transfer the chicken to the oven (if pan is not ovenproof place it in a baking tray) and bake for 8 to 10 minutes or until it is cooked through.

Take the chicken out of the oven, cover with foil, and let it rest for five minutes before you serve.

Meanwhile, in a steamer, steam the kale for about 5 minutes.

In a little oil, fry the ginger and red onions until they are soft but not coloured, and then add in the cooked kale and fry it for a minute.

Cook the buckwheat in accordance to the packet directions with the remaining turmeric.

Serve alongside the vegetables, salsa and chicken.

Nutrition: Calories 213, Fat: 6g, Carbs: 7g, Protein: 22g

48. Sirt salmon salad

Preparation time: 5 minutes

Cooking time: 30 minutes

Servings: 3

Ingredients:

1 large Medjool date, pitted then chopped

Olive oil

Parsley

Celery leaves

Walnuts

Capers

Red onions-sliced

Smoked salmon slices

Directions:

Arrange all the salad leaves on a large plate then mix the rest of the ingredients and distribute evenly on top the leaves.

Nutrition: Calories 453, Fat: 4g, Carbs: 8g, Protein: 19g

49. Greek salad skewers

Preparation time: 5 minutes

Cooking time: 30 minutes

Servings: 3

Ingredients:

Cucumber

Tomatoes

Black olives

Red onion

Skewers

For the dressing:

Juice of ½ lemon

½ garlic clove, peeled and crushed

1 tablespoon of of extra virgin olive oil

A few leaves of finely chopped basil

Generous seasoning of salt and freshly ground black pepper a few finely chopped oregano leaves

1 teaspoon of of balsamic vinegar

Directions:

Thread every skewer with salad ingredients in this order; olive, followed by tomato, then yellow pepper, red onion, followed by cucumber then feta, tomato, olive, then yellow pepper, red onion and finally cucumber.

Place the dressing ingredients in a small bowl, mix them thoroughly, and then pour over the skewers.

Nutrition: Calories 209, Fat: 8g, Carbs: 8g, Protein: 21g

50. Mediterranean Chicken Breasts

Preparation time: 5 minutes

Cooking time: 1 hour 5 minutes

Servings: 2

Ingredients:

2 teaspoon of olive oil

1 medium lemon, sliced

½ lb chicken breasts, halved

Salt and black pepper to season

1 tablespoon of capers, rinsed

1 cup chicken broth

2 tablespoon of chopped fresh parsley, divided

Directions:

Lay a piece of parchment paper on a baking sheet. Preheat the oven to 350°F.

Lay the lemon slices on the baking sheet, drizzle them with olive oil and sprinkle with salt. Roast in the oven for 25 minutes to brown the lemon rinds.

Cover the chicken with plastic wrap, place them on a flat surface, and gently pound with the rolling pin to flatten to about ½ -inch thickness.

Remove the plastic wraps and season the chicken with salt and pepper; set aside.

Heat the olive oil in a skillet over medium heat and fry the chicken on both sides to a golden brown for about 8 minutes in total.

Then, pour the chicken broth in, shake the skillet, and let the broth boil and reduce to a thick consistency, about 12 minutes.

Lightly stir in capers, roasted lemon, black pepper, olive oil, and parsley; simmer on low heat for 10 minutes. Serve the chicken with the sauce and sprinkled with fresh parsley.

Nutrition: Calories 430, **Fat:** 23g, **Carbs:** 13g, **Protein:** 33g

51. Greek-Style Chicken with Olives & Capers

Preparation time: 5 minutes

Cooking time: 20 minutes

Servings: 2

Ingredients:

1 red onion, chopped

½ lb chicken breasts, skinless and boneless

2 garlic cloves, minced

1 tablespoon of capers

2 tomatoes, chopped

½ teaspoon of red chili flakes

Directions:

Warm olive oil in a skillet over medium heat and cook the chicken for 2 minutes per side. Sprinkle with black pepper and salt. Set the chicken breasts in the oven at 450°F and bake for 8 minutes. Arrange the chicken on a platter.

In the same pan over medium heat, add the onion, olives, capers, garlic, and chili flakes, and cook for 1 minute. Stir in the tomatoes, pepper, and salt, and cook for 2 minutes. Sprinkle over the chicken breasts and enjoy.

Nutrition: Calories 387, Fat: 21g, Carbs: 12g, Protein: 23g

52. Fried Cod with Celery Wine Sauce

Preparation time: 5 minutes

Cooking time: 15 minutes

Servings: 2

Ingredients:

2 teaspoon of extra-virgin olive oil

2 cod fillets

2 garlic cloves, minced

Juice of 1 lemon

3 tablespoon of white wine

1 stalk celery, chopped

1 small red onion, chopped

Salt and black pepper to taste

Directions:

Heat 2 tablespoon of of the oil in a skillet over medium heat and season the cod with salt and black pepper. Fry the fillets in the oil for 4 minutes on one side, flip and cook for 1 minute. Take out, plate, and set aside.

In another skillet over low heat, warm the remaining olive oil and sauté the garlic and celery for 3 minutes. Add the lemon juice, wine, and red onions. Season with salt, black pepper, and cook for 3 minutes until the wine slightly reduces.

Put the fish in the skillet, spoon sauce over, cook for 30 seconds, and turn the heat off. Divide fish into plates, top with sauce, and serve.

Nutritin: Calories 264, Fat: 17g, Carbs: 9g, Protein: 20g

53. Minty Pesto Rubbed Beef Tenderloins

Preparation time: 5 minutes

Cooking time: 3 hours 10 minutes

Servings: 1

Ingredients:

1 cup fresh parsley, roughly chopped

1 teaspoon of fresh mint

1 red onion, chopped

5 oz beef tenderloin

1 lemon zested and juiced

3 tablespoon of olive oil, divided

1 oz walnuts, chopped

Salt to taste

3 garlic cloves, minced

Directions:

Preheat oven to 360 F.

In a food processor, combine the parsley with 2 tablespoon of of olive oil, mint, garlic, walnuts, salt, lemon zest, and red onion. Rub the beef with the mixture, place in a bowl, and refrigerate for 1 hour covered.

Remove the beef and warm 1 tablespoon of of olive oil in a skillet over high heat. Sear the meat for 3 to 5 minutes, depending on how you like it done. Transfer to a baking dish and cook in the oven for 16 minutes. Serve with a salad.

Nutrition: Calories 528, Fat: 38g, Carbs: 23g, Protein: 37g

54. Crispy Salmon Shirataki Fettucine

Preparation time: 5 minutes

Cooking time: 30 minutes

Servings: 2

Ingredients:

For the shirataki fettuccine:

1 (4 oz) pack shirataki fettuccine

For the creamy salmon sauce:

3 tablespoon of extra-virgin olive oil

2 salmon fillets, cut into 2-inch cubes

Salt and black pepper to taste

3 garlic cloves, minced

1 cup heavy cream

½ cup dry white wine

1 teaspoon of grated lemon zest

1 cup baby spinach

Lemon wedges for garnishing

Directions:

For the shirataki fettuccine:

Boil 2 cups of water in a pot over medium heat. Strain the shirataki pasta through a colander and rinse very well under hot running water. Pour the shirataki pasta into the boiling water. Take off the heat, let sit for 3 minutes and strain again.

Place a dry skillet over medium heat and stir-fry the shirataki pasta until visibly dry, and makes a squeaky sound when stirred, 1 to 2 minutes. Take off the heat and set aside.

For the salmon sauce:

Melt half of the olive oil in a large skillet; season the salmon with salt, black pepper, and cook in the butter until golden brown on all sides and flaky within, 8 minutes. Transfer to a plate and set aside. Add the remaining olive oil to the skillet and stir in the garlic. Cook until fragrant, 1 minute.

Mix in heavy cream, white wine, lemon zest, salt, and pepper. Allow boiling over low heat for 5 minutes. Stir in spinach, allow wilting for 2 minutes and stir in shirataki fettuccine and salmon until well-coated in the sauce. Garnish with the lemon wedges.

Nutrition: Calories 473, Fat: 48g, Carbs: 21g, Protein: 25g

55. Parsley-Lime Shrimp Pasta

Preparation time: 5 minutes

Cooking time: 15 minutes

Servings: 4

Ingredients:

2 tablespoon of butter

1 lb jumbo shrimp, peeled and deveined

4 garlic cloves, minced

1 pinch red chili flakes

¼ cup white wine

1 lime, zested and juiced

3 medium zucchinis, spiralized

Salt and black pepper to taste

2 tablespoon of chopped parsley

1 cup grated Parmesan cheese for topping

Directions:

Melt the butter in a large skillet and cook the shrimp until starting to turn pink.

Flip and stir in the garlic and red chili flakes. Cook further for 1 minute or until the shrimp is pink and opaque. Transfer to a plate and set aside.

Pour the wine and lime juice into the skillet, and cook until reduced by a quarter. Meanwhile, stir to deglaze the bottom of the pot.

Mix in the zucchinis, lime zest, shrimp, and parsley. Season with salt and black pepper, and toss everything well. Cook until the zucchinis is slightly tender for 2 minutes. Dish the food onto serving plates and top generously with the Parmesan cheese.

Nutrition: Calories 315, Fat: 10g, Carbs: 43g, Protein: 27g

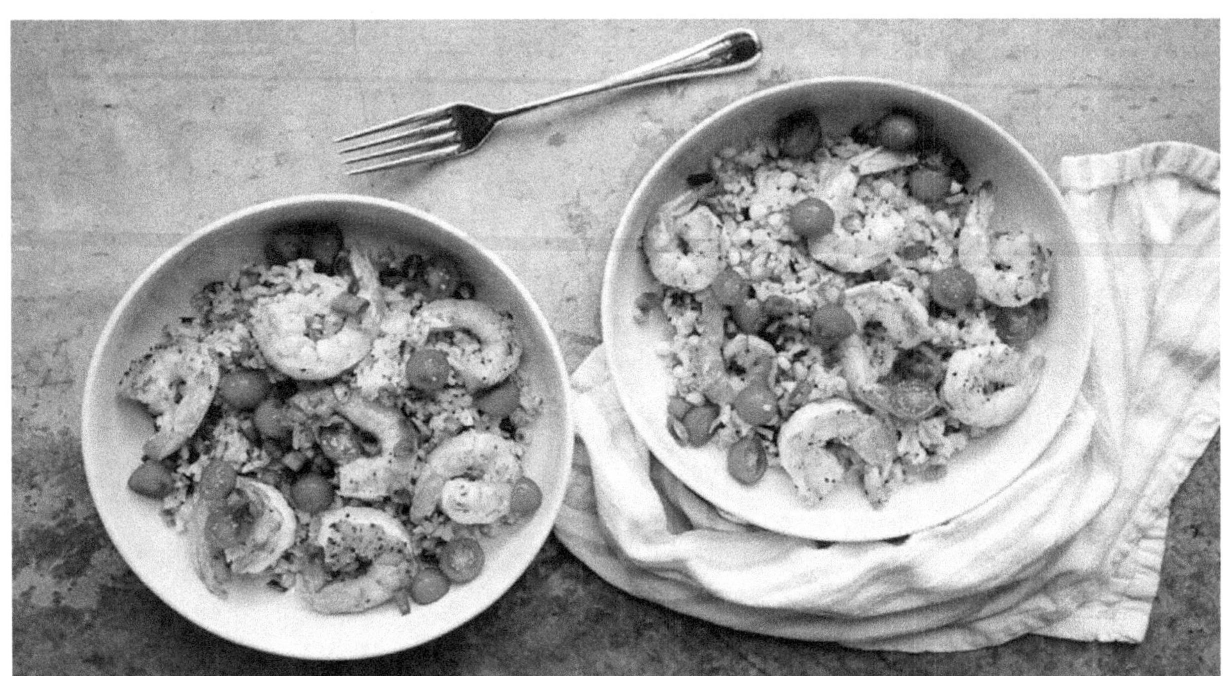

56. Green Goddess

Preparation Time: 15 minutes

Cooking Time: 1 hour 15 minutes

Servings: 8

Ingredients:

¾ cup sour cream

¾ cup mayonnaise

2 cloves garlic, minced

¼ cup fresh parsley leaves

2 teaspoon ofs. chopped fresh tarragon

1 tablespoon of. lemon juice

2 anchovy fillets

¼ cup minced fresh chives

Salt and ground black pepper to taste

Directions:

In a food processor or blender, process garlic, lemon juice, sour cream, anchovy fillets, parsley, tarragon, and mayonnaise until creamy and smooth.

Place the blended mixture in a bowl and stir in the minced chives gently. Season it with pepper and salt. Store it inside the refrigerator for at least 60 minutes before serving.

Nutrition: Calories 14, Fat: 2g, Carbs: 33g, Protein: 1g

57. Sage Carrots

Preparation Time: 10 minutes

Cooking Time: 30 minutes

Servings: 4

Ingredients:

2 teaspoon sweet paprika

1 tablespoon chopped sage

2 tablespoon olive oil

1 lb. peeled and roughly cubed carrots

¼ teaspoon black pepper

1 chopped red onion

Directions:

In a baking pan, combine the carrots with the oil and the other ingredients, toss and bake at 380 0F for 30 minutes.

Divide between plates and serve.

Nutrition: Calories 200, Fat: 3g, Carbs: 29g, Protein: 4g

58. Hearty Cashew and Almond Butter

Preparation Time: 5 minutes

Cooking Time: 12 minutes

Servings: 1

Ingredients:

1 cup almonds, blanched

⅓ cup cashew nuts

2 tablespoons coconut oil

½ teaspoon cinnamon

Directions:

Pre-heat your oven to 350 degrees F.

Bake almonds and cashews for 12 minutes.

Let them cool.

Transfer to food processor and add remaining ingredients.

Add oil and keep blending until smooth.

Serve and enjoy!

Nutrition: Calories 205, Fat: 6g, Carbs: 34g, Protein: 6g

59. Shrimp and Endives

Preparation Time: 5 minutes

Cooking Time: 12 minutes

Servings: 4

Ingredients:

1-pound shrimp, peeled and deveined

2 tablespoons avocado oil

2 spring onions, chopped

2 endives, shredded

1 tablespoon balsamic vinegar

1 tablespoon chives, minced

A pinch of sea salt and black pepper

Directions:

Heat up a pan with the oil over medium-high heat, add the spring onions, endives and chives, stir and cook for 4 minutes.

Add the shrimp and the rest of the ingredients, toss, cook over medium heat for 8 minutes more, divide into bowls and serve.

Nutrition: Calories 169, Fat: 2g, Carbs: 11g, Protein: 1g

60. Coriander Snapper Mix

Preparation Time: 5 minutes

Cooking Time: 20 minutes

Servings: 4

Ingredients:

2 tablespoons olive oil

2 garlic cloves, minced

4 snapper fillets, boneless, skinless and cubed

1 tomato, cubed

1 zucchini, cubed

1 tablespoon coriander, chopped

½ teaspoon cumin, ground

½ teaspoon rosemary, dried

A pinch of salt and black pepper

Directions:

Heat up a pan with the oil over medium-high heat, add the garlic, tomato and zucchini and cook for 5 minutes.

Add the fish and the other ingredients, toss, cook the mix for 15 minutes more, divide it into bowls and serve.

Nutrition: Calories 259, Fat: 4g, Carbs: 14g, Protein: 7g

61. Cherry Chicken Lettuce Wraps

Preparation Time: 15 minutes

Cooking Time: 10 minutes

Servings: 1

Ingredients:

12 lettuce leaves

2 tablespoon of canola oil, separated

⅓ cup sliced almonds, toasted

1 ¼ lb chicken breast, the skin and bones removed and minced

½ cup green onion, diced

1 tablespoon of fresh ginger root, thinly cut

1 ½ cups carrots, roughly cut

2 tablespoon of rice vinegar

1 lb. dark sweet cherries, cut in halves and the pits removed

2 tablespoon of teriyaki sauce

1 tablespoon of honey

Directions:

Set your stove to medium high heat and place a large sized skillet on it. Add 1 tablespoon of of oil to the pan and let it get hot. Put the skinless and boneless chicken in the pot and add your ginger. Sauté for 10 minutes. Be careful not to burn your chicken. You just want to make sure it is cooked through.

Get a bowl and add honey, vinegar, 1 tablespoon of oil, and teriyaki sauce. Using a whisk, mix these ingredients well, before throwing in your almonds, the chicken mixture in your skillet, green onion, cherries and carrots.

Using a spoon, place the mixture in the center of each of the twelve lettuce leaves. Roll the lettuce to cover this filling, and they are ready to serve.

Nutrition:

Calories 297, Fat: 12g, Carbs: 21g, Protein: 25g

62. Easy Korean Beef

Preparation Time: 10 minutes

Cooking Time: 10 minutes

Servings: 4

Ingredients:

1 tablespoon of sesame seeds

2 teaspoon of sesame oil

2 tablespoon of green onion, diced

1 lb. lean ground beef

2 cups cauliflower rice

3 garlic cloves, thinly cut

¼ teaspoon of ground black pepper

¼ cup soy sauce

¼ teaspoon of ground ginger

1 tablespoon of coconut sugar

Directions

Make sure your stove is set to medium high heat and place a large skillet on it. Pour the sesame oil in the pan to make it hot, before adding garlic and ground beef. After 7 minutes, by which time the beef would crumble easily, turn down the stove to low and quickly continue with the following step.

Grab a bowl and throw your black pepper, soy sauce, ginger, and coconut sugar in it. Using a whisk, mix these ingredients properly. Now, you can pour the coconut sugar mixture over the cooked beef that is still in the pan. Increase the heat back to medium and let the beef mixture simmer for about 3 minutes.

Serve the keto Korean beef on top of your prepared cauliflower rice. Finally, garnish with sesame seeds and green onions.

Nutrition: Calories 290, Fat: 13g, Carbs: 8g, Protein: 22g

63. Peanut Sesame Shirataki Noodles

Preparation Time: 20 minutes

Cooking Time: 10 minutes

Servings: 4

Ingredients:

1 8 oz pack shirataki noodles

2 tablespoon of creamy peanut butter

Snow peas

1 tablespoon of water

1 medium carrot, shredded

1 tablespoon of soy sauce, low sodium

Peanuts

1 teaspoon of rice vinegar

Toasted sesame seeds

Pinch garlic powder

Green onions

¼ teaspoon of black pepper

Cilantro

1 teaspoon of brown sugar

Pinch ground ginger

⅛ teaspoon of sesame oil

Directions:

Grab a medium sized bowl and put the ground ginger, peanut butter, sesame oil, water, brown sugar, soy sauce, black pepper, rice vinegar, and garlic powder inside it. Mix properly and set the bowl aside for 30 minutes.

Next, pop that bowl in the refrigerator until you have to use it on the pasta.

To prepare the pasta

Rinse your shirataki noodles. Follow that by draining the noodles and patting them dry using a paper towel.

Get a nonstick pan and place it over medium low heat. The pan has to be completely dry before the noodles. The purpose of this is to further make sure that the noodles are not wet. Do not burn them.

Chop your snow peas and add them, along with the grated carrots, into the pan containing your noodles. Sauté for about 4 minutes before you pour the sauce in. Mix the sauce into the other ingredients well.

Decorate with cilantro, toasted sesame seeds, green onions, and peanuts. Alternatively, you can choose to not garnish the meal.

Nutrition: Calories 119, Fat: 6g, Carbs: 9g, Protein: 12g

64. Ginger Asian Slaw

Preparation Time: 15 minutes

Cooking Time: 0 minutes

Servings: 8

Ingredients:

Sea salt to your preferred taste

6 cups Napa cabbage, minced

Pepper to your preferred taste

6 cups red cabbage, minced

3 tablespoon of lime juice

2 cups carrots grated

1 medium lime zest

1 cup cilantro, shredded

¼ teaspoon of cayenne pepper

¾ cup diced green onions

1 garlic clove, thinly cut

1 tablespoon of extra virgin olive oil

1 ½ inch ginger, shredded

1 tablespoon of maple syrup

2 tablespoon of almond butter

1 teaspoon of sesame oil

1 tablespoon of rice vinegar

1 tablespoon of apple cider vinegar

2 tablespoon of tamari

Directions:

Into the cup of a blender add your olive oil, salt, pepper, maple syrup, lime juice, sesame oil, lime zest, apple cider vinegar, cayenne pepper, tamari, garlic rice vinegar, ginger, and almond butter. Blend these ingredients until you are left with a smooth mixture. This is your dressing.

Next, you'll need a large mixing bowl. Put the cilantro, cabbage, green onions, and carrots inside it. Pour the mixture in your blender into the bowl and toss well.

For about an hour, let the bowl stay in your fridge. The various flavors will meld deliciously and afterwards, you can serve.

Nutrition: Calories 144, Fat: 6g, Carbs: 12g, Protein: 21g

Preparation Time: 10 minutes

Cooking Time: 25 minutes

Servings: 8

Ingredients:

4 cups vegetable stock

2 tablespoons olive oil

2 sweet potatoes, peeled and cubed

8 zucchinis, chopped

2 onions, peeled and chopped

1 cup coconut milk

A pinch of salt and black pepper

1 teaspoon dried rosemary

4 tablespoons fresh dill, chopped

½ teaspoon fresh basil, chopped

Directions:

Heat a pot with the oil over medium heat, add the onion, stir, and cook for 2 minutes. Add the zucchinis and the rest of the ingredients except the milk and dill, stir and simmer for 20 minutes.

Nutrition: Calories 324, Fat: 2g, Carbs: 10g, Protein: 14g

66. Masala Scallops

Preparation Time: 10 minutes

Cooking Time: 20 minutes

Servings: 4

Ingredients:

2 tablespoons olive oil

2 jalapenos, chopped

1-pound sea scallops

A pinch of salt and black pepper

¼ teaspoon cinnamon powder

1 teaspoon garam masala

1 teaspoon coriander, ground

1 teaspoon cumin, ground

2 tablespoons cilantro, chopped

Directions:

Heat up a pan with the oil over medium heat, add the jalapenos, cinnamon and the other ingredients except the scallops and cook for 10 minutes.

Add the rest of the ingredients, toss, cook for 10 minutes more, divide into bowls and serve.

Nutrition: Calories 281, Fat: 4g, Carbs: 11g, Protein: 17g

67. Tuna and Tomatoes

Preparation Time: 5 minutes

Cooking Time: 20 minutes

Servings: 4

Ingredients:

1 yellow onion, chopped

1 tablespoon olive oil

1-pound tuna fillets, boneless, skinless and cubed

1 cup tomatoes, chopped

1 red pepper, chopped

1 teaspoon sweet paprika

1 tablespoon coriander, chopped

Directions:

Heat up a pan with the oil over medium heat, add the onions and the pepper and cook for 5 minutes.

Add the fish and the other ingredients, cook everything for 15 minutes, divide between plates and serve.

Nutrition: Calories 159, Fat: 4g, Carbs: 14g, Protein: 7g

68. Scallops with Almonds and Mushrooms

Preparation Time: 5 minutes

Cooking Time: 10 minutes

Servings: 4

Ingredients:

1-pound scallops

2 tablespoons olive oil

4 scallions, chopped

½ cup mushrooms, sliced

2 tablespoon almonds, chopped

Directions:

Heat up a pan add the scallions and the mushrooms and sauté for 2 minutes.

Add the scallops and the other ingredients, toss, cook over medium heat for 8 minutes more, divide into bowls and serve.

Nutrition: Calories 322, Fat: 6g, Carbs: 8g, Protein: 21g

69. Ginger Mushrooms

Preparation Time: 10 minutes

Cooking Time: 20 minutes

Servings: 4

Ingredients:

1-pound mushrooms, sliced

1 yellow onion, chopped

1 tablespoon ginger, grated

1 tablespoon olive oil

2 tablespoons balsamic vinegar

2 garlic cloves, minced

A pinch of salt and black pepper

¼ cup lime juice

2 tablespoons walnuts, chopped

Directions:

Heat up a pan with the oil over medium-high heat, add the onion and the ginger and sauté for 5 minutes.

Add the mushrooms and the other ingredients, toss, cook over medium heat for 15 minutes more, divide between plates and serve.

Nutrition: Calories 129, Fat: 2g, Carbs: 4g, Protein: 5g

Preparation Time: 10 minutes

Cooking Time: 0 minutes

Servings: 4

Ingredients:

2 tablespoon ofs. olive oil

1 teaspoon of. dried rosemary

2 halved endives

¼ teaspoon of. black pepper

½ teaspoon of. turmeric powder

Directions:

In a baking pan, combine the endives with the oil and the other ingredients, toss gently, introduce in the oven and bake at 400 0F for 20 minutes.

Divide between plates and serve.

Nutrition: Calories 159, Fat: 2g, Carbs: 2g, Protein: 1g

71. Kale Sauté

Preparation Time: 10 minutes

Cooking Time: 10 minutes

Servings: 4

Ingredients:

1 chopped red onion

3 tablespoon ofs. Coconut amines

2 tablespoon ofs. olive oil

1 lb. torn kale

1 tablespoon of. chopped cilantro

1 tablespoon of. lime juice

2 minced garlic cloves

Directions:

Heat up a pan with the olive oil over medium heat, add the onion and the garlic and sauté for 5 minutes.

Add the kale and the other ingredients, toss, cook over medium heat for 10 minutes, divide between plates and serve.

Nutrition: Calories 200, Fat: 6g, Carbs: 6g, Protein: 6g

72. Roasted Beets

Preparation Time: 10 minutes

Cooking Time: 35 minutes

Servings: 2

Ingredients:

Garlic cloves

Black pepper

Beets

Walnuts

2 tablespoon ofs. olive oil

¼ c. chopped parsley

Directions:

In a baking dish, combine the beets with the oil and the other ingredients, toss to coat, introduce in the oven at 420 0F, and bake for 35 minutes.

Divide between plates and serve.

Nutrition: Calories 159, Fat: 6g, Carbs: 11g, Protein: 3g

73. Minty Tomatoes and Corn

Preparation Time: 5 minutes

Cooking Time: 0 minutes

Servings: 4

Ingredients:

2 c. corn

1 tablespoon of. rosemary vinegar

2 tablespoon ofs. chopped mint

1 lb. sliced tomatoes

¼ teaspoon of. black pepper

2 tablespoon ofs. olive oil

Directions:

In a salad bowl, combine the tomatoes with the corn and the other ingredients, toss and serve.

Enjoy!

Nutrition: Calories 200, Fat: 7g, Carbs: 11g, Protein: 2g

74. Pesto Green Beans

Preparation Time: 10 minutes

Cooking Time: 0 minutes

Servings: 4

Ingredients:

2 tablespoon ofs. olive oil

2 teaspoon ofs. sweet paprika

Juice of 1 lemon

2 tablespoon ofs. basil pesto

1 lb. trimmed and halved green beans

¼ teaspoon of. black pepper

1 sliced red onion

Directions:

Heat up a pan with the oil over medium-high heat, add the onion, stir and sauté for 5 minutes.

Add the beans and the rest of the ingredients, toss, cook over medium heat for 10 minutes, divide between plates and serve.

Nutrition: Calories 280, Fat: 3g, Carbs: 13g, Protein: 4g

75. Poached Eggs And Asparagus

Preparation time: 10 minutes

Cooking time: 10 minutes

Servings: 2

Ingredients:

4 eggs

1 cube chicken bouillon (optional)

1 pound fresh asparagus, trimmed

4 slices whole wheat bread

4 slices Cheddar cheese

1 tablespoon butter

salt and pepper to taste

Directions:

In a saucepan, fill half-way full of water. Boil and mix in bouillon cube until dissolved. Crack an egg into a large spoon or measuring cup and slip into boiling water gently. Repeat with the remaining eggs. Simmer over medium heat for 5 mins. Take out using a slotted spoon then keep it warm.

In the meantime, put asparagus into a saucepan and cover with enough water. Bring to a boil, cook for 4 mins or until the asparagus is tender. Drain.

Toast bread to your preferred darkness. Spread over each piece of toast with butter. Add one slice of cheese on top, then one poached egg and lastly, the asparagus. Add pepper and salt to taste. Enjoy right away!

Nutrition: Calories 306, Fat: 7g, Carbs: 18g, Protein: 18g

76. Red Curry Ham Gratin

Preparation time: 10 minutes

Cooking time: 20 minutes

Servings: 4

Ingredients:

1 ¼ cups whipping cream

¼ cup Greek yogurt

2 tablespoons red curry paste

1 tablespoon honey

1 pound spiral-sliced ham

2 ½ cups Yukon gold potatoes, thinly sliced

1 cup sliced leek

½ teaspoon salt

1 teaspoon ground black pepper, divided

2 cups shredded Monterey Jack cheese

1 green onion, thinly sliced

Directions

Set the oven to 350°F (175°C) and start preheating. Grease a 3-quart baking dish.

Stir honey, curry paste, yogurt and whipping cream together; pour ½ into the dish. Arrange leek, potatoes and ham in an overlapping layer; top with the rest of whipping cream mixture. Dust with cheese, ½ teaspoon pepper and salt.

Bake with an aluminum foil cover for 40 minutes. Uncover; keep baking for 20 more minutes until potatoes become tender and top turns golden brown. Let rest for 15 minutes. Decorate with the rest of black pepper and green onion.

Nutrition: Calories 359, Fat: 12g, Carbs: 18g, Protein: 21g

77. Zucchini Pancakes

Preparation Time: 15 minutes

Cooking Time: 8 minutes

Serving: 8

Ingredients:

12 tablespoons water

6 large zucchinis, grated

Sea salt, to taste

4 tablespoons ground Flax Seeds

2 teaspoons olive oil

2 jalapeño peppers, finely chopped

½ cup scallions, finely chopped

Directions:

Mix together water and flax seeds in a bowl and keep aside.

Heat oil in a large non-stick skillet on medium heat and add zucchini, salt, and black pepper.

Cook for about 3 minutes and transfer the zucchini into a large bowl. Stir in scallions and flax seed mixture and thoroughly mix.

Preheat a griddle and grease it lightly with cooking spray. Pour about ¼ of the zucchini mixture into preheated griddle and cook for about 3 minutes.

Flip the side carefully and cook for about 2 more minutes. Repeat with the remaining mixture in batches and serve.

Nutrition: Calories 132, Fat: 3g, Carbs: 9g, Protein: 4g

78. Squash Hash

Preparation Time: 2 minutes

Cooking Time: 10 minutes

Serving: 2

Ingredients:

1 teaspoon onion powder

½ cup onion, finely chopped

2 cups spaghetti squash

½ teaspoon sea salt

Directions:

Squeeze any extra moisture from spaghetti squash using paper towels. Place the squash into a bowl, then add the onion powder, onion, and salt. Stir to combine.

Spray a non-stick cooking skillet with cooking spray and place it over medium heat.

Add the spaghetti squash to pan. Cook the squash for 5 minutes, untouched. Using a spatula, flip the hash browns. Cook for an additional 5 minutes or until the desired crispness is reached. Serve and Enjoy!

Nutrition: Calories 180, Fat: 2g, Carbs: 8g, Protein: 1g

79. Carrots and Onion Mix

Preparation time: 10 minutes

Cooking time: 25 minutes

Servings: 4

Ingredients:

1 pound baby carrots, trimmed

3 garlic cloves, minced

1 cup pearl onions, peeled

Salt and black pepper to the taste

2 tablespoons coconut oil, melted

2 tablespoons chopped tarragon

¼ cup chopped parsley

Juice of 1 lemon

1 tablespoon chopped thyme

1 cup cherry tomatoes, halved

Directions:

Heat up a pan with the oil over medium-high heat, add the onions and garlic and cook for 5 minutes.

Add the rest of the ingredients, stir, cook for 20 minutes more, divide between plates and serve.

Nutrition: Calories 173, Fat: 3g, Carbs: 9g, Protein: 5g

80. Mixed Berry Crisp

Preparation Time: 10 Minutes

Cooking Time: 0

Servings: 4

Ingredients:

1 1/2 cups mixed berries (I used raspberries, blueberries and blackberries)

1/2 tablespoon cornstarch

2 tablespoons butter, room temperature

1/4 cup old fashioned oats, plus 1 tablespoon old fashioned oats

1/4 cup brown sugar

3 tablespoons flour

1/4 teaspoon cinnamon

1/4 teaspoon nutmeg

1 tablespoon water

Directions:

Preheat oven to 375 degrees.

In a small bowl, combine the butter, oats, brown sugar, flour, cinnamon and nutmeg. Mix lightly with a fork until the mixture is crumbly.

Top the berries with the crisp mixture. Sprinkle the top of the crisp with water.

Bake for 25 minutes or until the fruit is bubbling and the topping is slightly browned.

Serve with ice cream, frozen yogurt or whipped cream.

Nutrition: Calories 226, Fat: 21g, Carbs: 18g, Protein: 11g

81. Strawberry Daiquiri

Preparation Time: 10 Minutes

Cooking Time: 24 Minutes

Servings: 4

Ingredients:

1 (10 ounce) can froze strawberry daiquiri concentrate

1 (10 ounce) can froze strawberry daiquiri concentrate

1 1/2 cups frozen strawberries

1 cup ice cube

Directions:

Combine all ingredients together in blender until all the ice is crushed.

Add more or less ice-cubes for the right texture.

Nutrition: Calories 116, Fat: 21g, Carbs: 8g, Protein: 4g

82. Virgin White Sangria

Preparation Time: 5 Minutes

Cooking Time: 4 Minutes

Servings: 1

Ingredients:

Fresh fruit

 Lemon-lime soda

Directions:

Combine all the ingredients except the soda in a large pitcher and chill for at least 1 hour.

When serving, add the soda. Serve with a pretty fruit garnish.

Nutrition: Calories 129, Fat: 23g, Carbs: 8g, Protein: 18g

83.   Wow Cola Chicken

Preparation Time: 15 Minutes

Cooking Time: 14 Minutes

Servings: 1

Ingredients:

16 ounces boneless chicken breasts

 1 (12 ounce) can diet cola

 1 cup ketchup

Directions:

Place chicken in crockpot and then top with ketchup and then pour cola over all.

Cook on low for 6-8 hours.

Nutrition: Calories 218, Fat: 19g, Carbs: 18g, Protein: 28g

Preparation Time: 5 Minutes

Cooking Time: 4 Minutes

Servings: 1

Ingredients:

2 red apples, cored & cut in half

1 (375 ml) canflavoured diet cola (cherry or strawberry suggested)

1 pinch Splenda sugar substitute or 1 pinch Equal sugar substitute

1 pinch cinnamon

Directions:

Place the apple in a baking dish, skin side down and pour the cola over.

Sprinkle with sweetener & cinnamon.

Bake in a pre-heated oven at 180.C for 25-30 minutes.

Nutrition: Calories 156, Fat: 22g, Carbs: 5g, Protein: 4g

Preparation Time: 5 minutes

Cooking Time: 10 minutes

Serving: 2

Ingredients:

1 bell pepper, any color, seeded and sliced

Juice of ½ a lime

2 tablespoons fresh cilantro

½ teaspoon cumin

1 teaspoon sea salt

1 jalapeno, chopped

½ cup zucchini, sliced

1 cup cherry tomatoes, halved

½ cup mushrooms, sliced

1 cup broccoli florets, cooked

1 sweet onion, chopped

Directions:

Spray a non-stick pan with cooking spray and place it over medium heat.

Add the onion, broccoli, bell pepper, tomatoes, zucchini, mushrooms and jalapeno. Cook for 7 minutes, or until desired doneness is reached. Stir occasionally.

Stir in the cumin, cilantro, and salt. Cook for 3 minutes while stirring.

Remove pan from heat, then add the lime juice.

Divide between serving plates, serve and enjoy!

Nutrition: Calories 90, Fat: 2g, Carbs: 16g, Protein: 4g

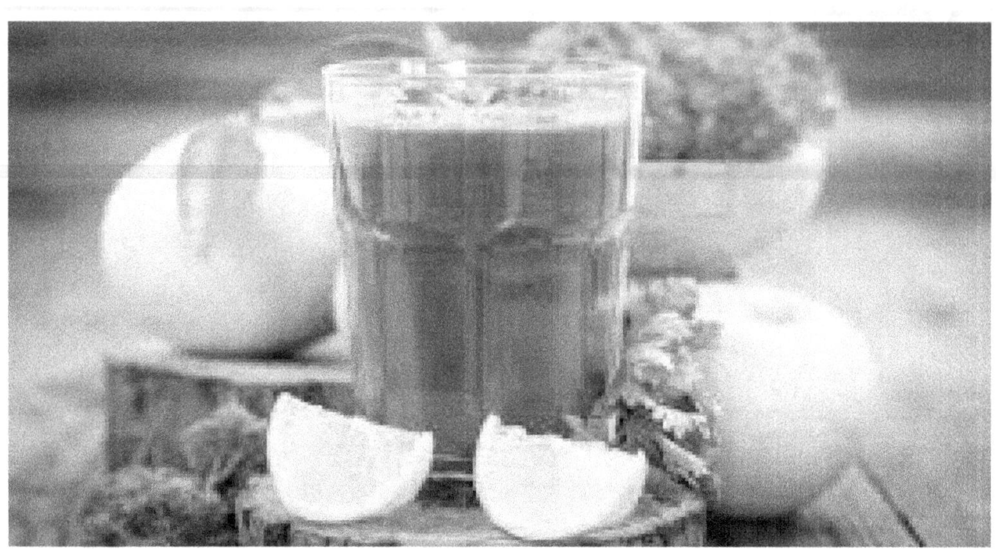

86. Kale Kiwi Smoothie

Preparation Time: 10 minutes

Cooking Time: 5 minutes

Servings: 1

Ingredients:

1 cup Kale, chopped

2 Apples

3 Kiwis

1 tablespoon flax seeds

1 tablespoon royal jelly

1 cup crushed ice

Directions:

Place all of the ingredients into a blender and cover them with water. You can also add some crushed ice and a mint leaf to garnish.

Nutrition: Calories 145, Fat: 6g, Carbs: 17g, Protein: 9g

87. Salad Smoothie

Preparation Time: 10 minutes

Cooking Time: 5 minutes

Servings: 1

Ingredients:

1 cup arugula

½ cucumber

Red onion

Parsley

Lemon juice

Crushed ice

Olive oil

Directions:

Put all the ingredients into a blender with some water until smooth. Add ice to make your smoothie refreshing.

Nutrition: Calories 108, Fat: 2g, Carbs: 14g, Protein: 6g

88. Avocado Kale Smoothie

Preparation Time: 10 minutes

Cooking Time: 5 minutes

Servings: 1

Ingredients:

1 cup Kale

½ Avocado

1 cup Cucumber

1 Celery Stalk

1 tablespoon of. chia seeds

1 cup crushed ice

1 tablespoon of. Spirulina

Directions:

Place all of the ingredients into a blender and add in enough water to cover them. Process until smooth, serve and enjoy.

Nutrition: Calories 159, Fat: 2g, Carbs: 8g, Protein: 4g

89. Kale Banana Apple Smoothie

Preparation Time: 10 minutes

Cooking Time: 5 minutes

Servings: 1

Ingredients:

1 cup Kale

2 Apples

¾ avocado

1 banana

1 tablespoon of.

1 cup crushed ice

Directions:

Place all of the ingredients into a blender and process until smooth. Serve and enjoy.

Nutrition: Calories 132, Fat: 4g, Carbs: 8g, Protein: 10g

90. Kale Cucumber Apple Smoothie

Preparation Time: 10 minutes

Cooking Time: 5 minutes

Servings: 1

Ingredients:

1 cup Kale

2 Apples

1 avocado

1 Lime

¼ cup Raspberries

1 Cucumber

1 cup crushed ice

Directions:

Place all of the ingredients into blender with enough water to cover them.

Nutrition: Calories 134, Fat: 5g, Carbs: 8g, Protein: 4g

91. Grapefruit Kale Smoothie

Preparation Time: 10 minutes

Cooking Time: 5 minutes

Servings: 1

Ingredients:

1 large grapefruit

1 Apple

1 cup watercress

2 Kale leaves

1 Tablespoon of. dill (optional)

1 cup crushed ice

Directions:

Place all of the ingredients into a blender and add enough water to cover them. Process until creamy and smooth.

Nutrition: Calories 213, Fat: 4g, Carbs: 8g, Protein: 4g

92. Pear Cilantro Smoothie

Preparation Time: 10 minutes

Cooking Time: 5 minutes

Servings: 1

Ingredients:

1 cup Parsley leaves

1 pear

¾ avocado

½ lemon - juice

1 tablespoon of. chopped Cilantro

1 cup crushed ice

Directions:

Place all of the ingredients into a blender with enough water to cover them and process until smooth. Add a few ice cubes and enjoy.

Nutrition: Calories 349, Fat: 6g, Carbs: 6g, Protein: 8g

93. Kale Avocado Smoothie

Preparation Time: 10 minutes

Cooking Time: 5 minutes

Servings: 1

Ingredients:

1 cup Strawberries

1 cup Kale

½ avocado

½ lemon

1 cup crushed ice

Directions:

Place all of the ingredients into a blender with enough water to cover them and process until smooth. Add a few ice cubes and enjoy.

Nutrition: Calories 340, Fat: 4g, Carbs: 6g, Protein: 9g

94. Kale, Parsley and Banana Smoothie

Preparation Time: 10 minutes

Cooking Time: 5 minutes

Servings: 1

Ingredients:

1 cup chopped kale

2 bananas

½ cup chopped parsley

1 tablespoon of.

1 cup crushed ice

Directions:

Place all of the ingredients into a blender with enough water to cover them and process until smooth. Add a few ice cubes and enjoy.

Nutrition: Calories 334, Fat: 4g, Carbs: 8g, Protein: 4g

95. Kefir Kale Banana Orange Chia Smoothie

Preparation Time: 10 minutes

Cooking Time: 5 minutes

Servings: 1

Ingredients:

½ Orange

1 banana

1 cup Kale

¼ cup chia seeds

½ cup kefir

1 cup crushed ice

Directions:

Place all of the ingredients into a blender with enough water to cover them and process until smooth. Add a few ice cubes and enjoy.

Nutrition: Calories 359, Fat: 4g, Carbs: 12g, Protein: 9g

96. Green Tea Smoothie

Preparation time: 20 Minutes

Cooking Time: 0 Minutes

Servings: 2

Ingredients:

2 teaspoons of honey

250 ml of milk

2 teaspoons of matcha green tea powder 6 ice cubes

½ teaspoon of vanilla bean paste not extractor a scrape of the seeds from the vanilla pod

2 ripe bananas

Directions:

Place all the ingredients in a blender and run until you achieve the desired consistency.

Serve into two glasses and enjoy.

Nutrition: Calories 180, Fat: 1g, Carbs: 5g, Protein: 2g

97. Berries Banana Smoothie

Preparation time: 10 Minutes

Cooking Time: 0 Minutes

Servings: 2

Ingredients:

½ cup of coconut milk

1½ cups of mixed berries strawberries and blueberries) - could be frozen or fresh

¾ cup of water

4 ice cubes

1 tablespoon of molasses

1 banana

Directions:

Place all the ingredients in a blender and blend until smooth.

You can add water to the smoothie until you achieve your desired consistency, then serve.

Nutrition: Calories 112, Fat: 6g, Carbs: 29g, Protein: 9g

98. Mango & Rocket Arugula Smoothie

Preparation time: 10 Minutes

Cooking Time: 0 Minutes

Servings: 2

Ingredients:

25g 1ozfresh rocket arugula

150g 5ozfresh mango, peeled, de-stoned and chopped

1 avocado, de-stoned and peeled

Directions:

Place all of the ingredients into a blender with enough water to cover them and process until smooth. Add a few ice cubes and enjoy.

Nutrition: Calories 188, Fat: 6g, Carbs: 18g, Protein: 10g

99. Grape and Melon Smoothie

Preparation time: 20 Minutes

Cooking Time: 0 Minutes

Servings: 1

Ingredients:

100g of cantaloupe melon

100g of red seedless grapes

30g of young spinach leaves stalks removed

½ cucumber

Directions:

Peel the cucumber, then cut it into half. Remove the seeds and chop them roughly.

Peel the cantaloupe, deseed it, and cut it into chunks.

Place all ingredients in a blender and blend until smooth.

Nutrition: Calories 342, Fat: 1g, Carbs: 3g, Protein: 6g

100.   Matcha Green Tea Smoothie

Preparation time: 10 Minutes

Cooking Time: 0 Minutes

Servings: 2

Ingredients:

2 bananas

2 teaspoon Matcha green tea powder

½ teaspoon vanilla bean paste

1 ½ cups milk

4-5 ice cubes

2 teaspoon honey

Directions:

Add all ingredients except the Matcha to a blender. Blend until smooth. Sprinkle in the Matcha tea powder, stir well or blend a few seconds more or add cooled green tea.

Nutrition: Calories 342, Fat: 2g, Carbs: 21g, Protein: 9g

101. Green-Berry Smoothie

Preparation time: 20 Minutes

Cooking Time: 0 Minutes

Servings: 2

Ingredients:

1 ripe banana

½ cup blackcurrants take off stems

10 baby kale leaves take off stems

2 teaspoon honey

1 cup freshly made green tea dissolve honey

6 ice cubes

Directions:

Dissolve the honey in the tea before you chill it. Cool first, and then blend all ingredients blender until smooth.

Nutrition: Calories 112, Fat: 6g, Carbs: 29g, Protein: 8g

102.   Creamy Strawberry & Cherry Smoothie

Preparation time: 20 Minutes

Cooking Time: 0 Minutes

Servings: 2

Ingredients:

100g 3½ oz. strawberries

75g 3oz. frozen pitted cherries

1 tablespoon plain full-fat yogurt

175mls 6fl oz. unsweetened soya milk

Directions:

Place all of the ingredients into a blender and process until smooth. Serve and enjoy.

Nutrition: Calories 132, Fat: 3g, Carbs: 39g, Protein: 9g

103.   Mango Smoothie

Preparation Time: 5 Minutes

Cooking Time: 0 minutes

Servings: 3

Ingredients:

1 Carrot, Peeled & Chopped

1 Cup Strawberries

1 Cup Water

1 Cup Peaches, Chopped

1 Banana, Frozen & sliced

1 Cup Mango, Chopped

Directions:

Blend everything together until smooth.

Nutrition: Calories 221, Fat: 1g, Carbs: 5g, Protein: 4g

104.   Spinach Peach Banana Smoothie

Preparation Time: 10 minutes

Cooking Time: 0 minutes

Servings: 2

Ingredients:

1 cup baby spinach

2 cups coconut water

1 tablespoon agave syrup

2 ripe bananas

2 ripe peaches, pitted and chopped

Directions:

Add all ingredients to the blender and blend until smooth and creamy.

Serve immediately and enjoy.

Nutrition: Calories 163, Fat: 1g, Carbs: 4g, Protein: 6g

Preparation Time: 10 minutes

Cooking Time: 0 minutes

Servings: 2

Ingredients:

1 cup ice cubes

¼ tablespoon liquid aminos

1 and ½ tablespoon sea salt

2 limes, peeled and quartered

1 avocado, pitted and peeled

1 cup kale leaves

1 cucumber, chopped

2 cups tomato, chopped

¼ cup water

Directions:

Add all ingredients to the blender and blend until smooth and creamy.

Serve immediately and enjoy.

Nutrition: Calories 108, Fat: 1g, Carbs: 1g, Protein: 4g

106.   Watermelon Strawberry Smoothie

Preparation Time: 10 minutes

Cooking Time: 0 minutes

Servings: 2

Ingredients:

1 cup coconut milk yogurt

½ cup strawberries

2 cups fresh watermelon

1 banana

Directions:

Toss in all your ingredients into your blender then process until smooth.

Serve and Enjoy.

Nutrition: Calories 160, Fat: 1g, Carbs: 3g, Protein: 4g

107.   Watermelon Kale Smoothie

Preparation Time: 10 minutes

Cooking Time: 0 minutes

Servings: 2

Ingredients:

8 oz water

1 orange, peeled

3 cups kale, chopped

1 banana, peeled

2 cups watermelon, chopped

1 celery, chopped

Directions:

Add all ingredients to the blender and blend until smooth and creamy.

Serve immediately and Enjoy.

Nutrition: Calories 122, Fat: 1g, Carbs: 5g, Protein: 1g

108.   Mix Berry Watermelon Smoothie

Preparation Time: 10 minutes

Cooking Time: 0 minutes

Servings: 2

Ingredients:

1 cup alkaline water

2 fresh lemon juices

¼ cup fresh mint leaves

1 and ½ cup mixed berries

2 cups watermelon

Directions:

Toss in all your ingredients into your blender then process until smooth. Serve immediately and Enjoy.

 Nutrition: Calories 188, Fat: 1g, Carbs: 2g, Protein: 1g

109.   Healthy Green Smoothie

Preparation Time: 10 minutes

Cooking Time: 0 minutes

Servings: 3

Ingredients:

1 cup water

1 fresh lemon, peeled

1 avocado

1 cucumber, peeled

1 cup spinach

1 cup ice cubes

Directions:

Add all ingredients to the blender and blend until smooth and creamy.

Serve immediately and enjoy.

Nutrition: Calories: 160, Fat: 13g, Carbs: 12g, Protein: 2g

110.   Apple Spinach Cucumber Smoothie

Preparation Time: 10 minutes

Cooking Time: 0 minutes

Servings: 1

Ingredients:

¾ cup water

½ green apple, diced

¾ cup spinach

½ cucumber

Directions:

Add all ingredients to the blender and blend until smooth and creamy.

Serve immediately and enjoy.

Nutrition: Calories: 90, Fat: 1g, Carbs: 21g, Protein: 1g

Preparation Time: 10 minutes

Cooking Time: 0 minutes

Servings: 2

Ingredients:

1 cup ice cubes

20 drops liquid stevia

2 fresh lime, peeled and halved

1 tablespoon lime zest, grated

½ cucumber, chopped

1 avocado, pitted and peeled

2 cups spinach

1 tablespoon creamed coconut

¾ cup coconut water

Directions:

Add all ingredients to the blender and blend until smooth and creamy.

Serve immediately and enjoy.

Nutrition: Calories 312, Fat: 3g, Carbs: 28g, Protein: 4g

112.   Broccoli Green Smoothie

Preparation Time: 10 minutes

Cooking Time: 0 minutes

Servings: 2

Ingredients:

1 celery, peeled and chopped

1 lemon, peeled

1 apple, diced

1 banana

1 cup spinach

½ cup broccoli

Directions:

Add all ingredients to the blender and blend until smooth and creamy.

Serve immediately and enjoy.

 Nutrition: Calories 121, Fat: 1g, Carbs: 18g, Protein: 1g

113.	Irish Coffee

Preparation time: 15 minutes

Cooking time: 0 minutes

Servings: 1

Ingredients:

1.5 cl of cane sugar syrup (or 2 pieces of sugar)

2 cl of fresh cream

4 cl of coffee

3 cl of whiskey (bourbon, whiskey)

Directions:

Make the "Irish Coffee" recipe directly in the glass.

Heat the whiskey with the sugar (at low heat so as not to boil the whiskey) in a saucepan stirring. Prepare a black coffee and pour it over the hot and sweet whiskey, stir slightly. Pour everything into the previously rinsed glass with warm water and coat the surface with lightly beaten cream, its ready! Savor without delay. To make your cream work better, place it in the freezer for 20 minutes before vigorously whipping it.

Despite some rumors of modern times, Irish coffee is not supposed to have the three separate floors. Other variants can be made with whipped cream instead of fresh cream, liquid cane sugar instead of powdered sugar or replace the traditional whiskey with whiskey or bourbon. Still, the original recipe is the one explained above.

Serve in a glass type "mug."

Add any grated chocolate to the cream.

Nutrition: Calories 189, Fat: 2g, Carbs: 4g, Protein: 15g

114.   Caramel Coffee

Preparation time: 15 minutes

Cooking time: 0 minutes

Servings: 1

Ingredients:

15 cl of milk

3 cl of caramel syrup

1 dash of cinnamon syrup

1 coffee

Directions:

Make the recipe "Coffee Caramel."

Make a coffee (espresso). Heat the glass under hot water and pour the caramel syrup into the bottom of the glass. Heat the milk in another container until creamy foam and pour the warm milk gently on the syrup. Pour a few drops of cinnamon syrup and pour the coffee gently over the milk (use a spoon) until you get an extra layer.

Serve in a tumbler type glass.

Sprinkle with cinnamon powder.

Nutrition: Calories 321, Fat: 4g, Carbs: 6g, Protein: 8g

115.   Latte Macchiato

Preparation time: 15 minutes

Cooking time: 0 minutes

Servings: 1

Ingredients:

Coffee

20 cl of milk

Directions:

Make the recipe "Latte macchiato" directly in the glass.

Beat the milk (preferably whole) with a whisk in a saucepan over the heat to obtain foam on the surface (or using the steam nozzle of your espresso machine).

Pour warm milk into a heat-resistant glass (thick walls), blocking the foam with a spatula.

Add the milk foam on the hot milk.

Finally, gently pour a strong espresso (sweetened according to taste) on the frothed milk.

Since whole milk has a higher density than espresso, the latter will be placed above the milk.

Serve in a tumbler type glass.

To serve, you can fill the milk foam with chocolate flakes, liquid caramel, cocoa powder, cinnamon or other spices.

Nutrition: Calories 129, Fat: 6g, Carbs: 29g, Protein: 6g

116.　　Latte Macchiato Caramel

Preparation time: 15 minutes

Cooking time: 0 minutes

Servings: 6

Ingredients:

1 l of milk

20 cl of coffee

10 cl of caramel syrup Directions:

Directions:

Make the recipe "Latte Macchiato Caramel" in the pan.

Heat the milk and prepare 20 cl of hot black coffee. Divide the milk into 4 large glasses and froth the milk with an emulsifier, electric whisk, or steam nozzle on your coffee maker until you have 2 to 3 cm of milk foam.

Pour about 2cl of caramel syrup into each glass and slowly pour 5cl of coffee.

The coffee will come just below the foam of milk, to form 3 layers: the milk at the bottom, the coffee, and the milk froth above.

Serve in a cup-type glass.

Pour a little caramel syrup over the milk foam.

Nutrition: Calories 223, Fat: 6g, Carbs: 18g, Protein: 9g

117.   Coffee Cream with Caramel Milk Foam

Preparation time: 15 minutes

Cooking time: 0 minutes

Servings: 4

Ingredients:

Grand Cru Volluto capsule (to prepare 40 ml of Espresso coffee)

100 ml of milk to prepare milk foam

Teaspoon caramel syrup

25 ml / 5 teaspoons of cream (already prepared or homemade according to the method indicated below)

For the preparation of 250 ml of homemade cream:

250 ml semi-skimmed milk

2 egg yolks

50 g of white sugar

Half vanilla pod cut lengthwise

Materials

Espresso Cup (80 Ml)

Directions:

Bring the milk to a boiling point along with half a vanilla pod in a casserole dish

Beat the egg yolks inside a bowl with the sugar

Continue beating the yolks and sugar while adding the milk with the half vanilla pod

Then, put the mixture back in the pan and let it thicken over low heat (do not let the mixture boil to prevent it from cutting)

Check the consistency of the cream with a spoon and, as soon as the cream begins to adhere to the spoon, remove the pan from the heat

Keep stirring the mixture to keep it soft and creamy

Take out the vanilla bean, scrape it with a knife to remove the seeds and put it back in the cream

Prepare a Volluto (25 ml) in an Espresso cup or a small Nespresso recipe glass and add 25 ml / five teaspoons of the homemade cream or ready-made cream

Prepare milk foam with the steam nozzle of your Espresso machine and add the caramel syrup as soon as the foam begins to form

Cover the coffee cream with the caramel-flavored milk foam and serve immediately

Nutrition: Calories 286, Fat: 2g, Carbs: 2g, Protein: 1g

118.   Hot and Cold Vanilla Espresso with Caramel Foam and Cookies

Preparation time: 15 minutes

Cooking time: 15 minutes

Servings: 4

Ingredients:

For hot and cold vanilla coffee:

Two capsules of Grand Cru Volluto

A scoop of vanilla ice cream

Three tablespoons of milk foam

Two teaspoons of caramel liquid

For the cookies:

70 g softened butter

70 g of sugar

Teaspoon honey

Egg

100 g flour

A pinch of salt

50 g grated chocolate

For hazelnut caramel:

50 g whole hazelnuts

40 g of sugar

Two tablespoons of water

Directions:

For hot and cold vanilla coffee:

Prepare the milk foam, add the liquid caramel, and reserve it

Prepare two coffees in a large cup and pour them into a cold glass

Add the vanilla ice cream ball immediately and cover it with the milk foam

For cookies:

- Preheat oven to 150 ° C

Heat sugar and water until caramelized, remove from heat and add crushed hazelnuts

Place the hazelnuts on a sheet of vegetable paper and roast them in the oven for 10 min, moving them occasionally

Put the butter, sugar, salt, honey and egg in a large bowl

Beat it all for a few seconds until you get a smooth mixture

Add caramelized hazelnuts and grated chocolate

Raise the oven temperature to 180 ° C

Put small balls of dough on the baking sheet lined with vegetable paper and bake for about 15 min

Let them cool on a rack.

Nutrition: Calories 186, Fat: 11g, Carbs: 2g, Protein: 9g

119.   Espresso with Cottage Cheese, Lime and Brazil Nuts

Preparation time: 5 minutes

Cooking time: 20 minutes

Servings: 6

Ingredients:

1 capsule of Grand Cru Volluto or Volluto Decaffeinato

550 g cottage cheese

100 g of sugar

The juice of a lime

2 egg whites

3 jelly sheets or a teaspoon of agar

80 g of Brazil nuts

Directions:

Roast the Brazil nuts in a pan and mash them finely.

Book them.

Dip the jelly leaves in cold water to soften them.

Grate and squeeze the file.

Boil 100 ml of water with sugar and lime juice for 5 minutes.

Remove from heat and add the drained gelatin and lime zest.

Beat the egg whites and mount them until stiff.

Pour three-quarters of the lime syrup over the egg whites without stopping to beat and then add the cottage cheese to the mixture.

Divide the crushed nuts into the six molds and cover them using a cottage cheese mousse.

Pour the remaining lime syrup over and put the molds in the refrigerator for 4 hours.

Serve it with a Grand Cru Volluto.

Nutrition: Calories 188, Fat: 6g, Carbs: 5g, Protein: 8g

120. Coffee with Malice

Preparation time: 5 minutes

Cooking time: 5 minutes

Servings: 4

Ingredients:

1 intense espresso coffee sachet

1 splash whiskey

1 splash whole milk or cream

Directions:

You can use the dolce gusto machine, but if you don't have one, you can do it with a good quality soluble coffee loaded. All right; Put the coffee sachet in the coffee maker and select the amount of water to pour.

Activate the hot water until it stops. Have whiskey on hand.

Pour a little squirt of whiskey, heat a little cream or milk, and add it to coffee.

Ready, you can add sugar or sweetener if it's your taste. I prefer it as it is. With its bitter touch.

Nutrition: Calories 394, Fat: 9g, Carbs: 17g, Protein: 10g

121.   Viennese Coffee

Preparation time: 5 minutes

Cooking time: 0 minutes

Servings: 1

Ingredients:

Espresso coffee to your liking.

Whole milk (if you are in full operation bikini, skimmed)

White sugar

Whipped cream

Shavings chocolate

Directions:

Take the coffee capsule. You put it in the machine and let it do its job.

You fill the glass of milk, add your healthy dose of sugar, and stir.

Decorate with a good tuft of cream and chocolate chips.

As you can see, very, very difficult to do. Having just spent the day.

Nutrition: Calories 259, Fat: 12g, Carbs: 4g, Protein: 2g

122.   Coffee Mousse

Preparation time: 5 minutes

Cooking time: 0 minutes

Servings: 6

Ingredients:

4 sheets jelly

125 ml of espresso coffee

2 tablespoons. Baileys

100 gr. sugar

Two egg whites

200 ml 35% mg whipping cream

Directions:

We put into hydrating the gelatin.

We prepare a coffee.

We ride the egg whites with the sugar about to snow.

We semi-cream.

Melt the jello in the hot coffee and add the Baileys.

Add the coffee to tablespoons to the whites mounted.

Add the whipped cream.

We pour the mixture into 6 glasses that we can decorate with sprinkled cocoa powder. In my case, I prepared a coffee jelly.

Let cool inside the fridge for a few hours and go!

Nutrition: Calories 123, Fat: 6g, Carbs: 4g, Protein: 8g

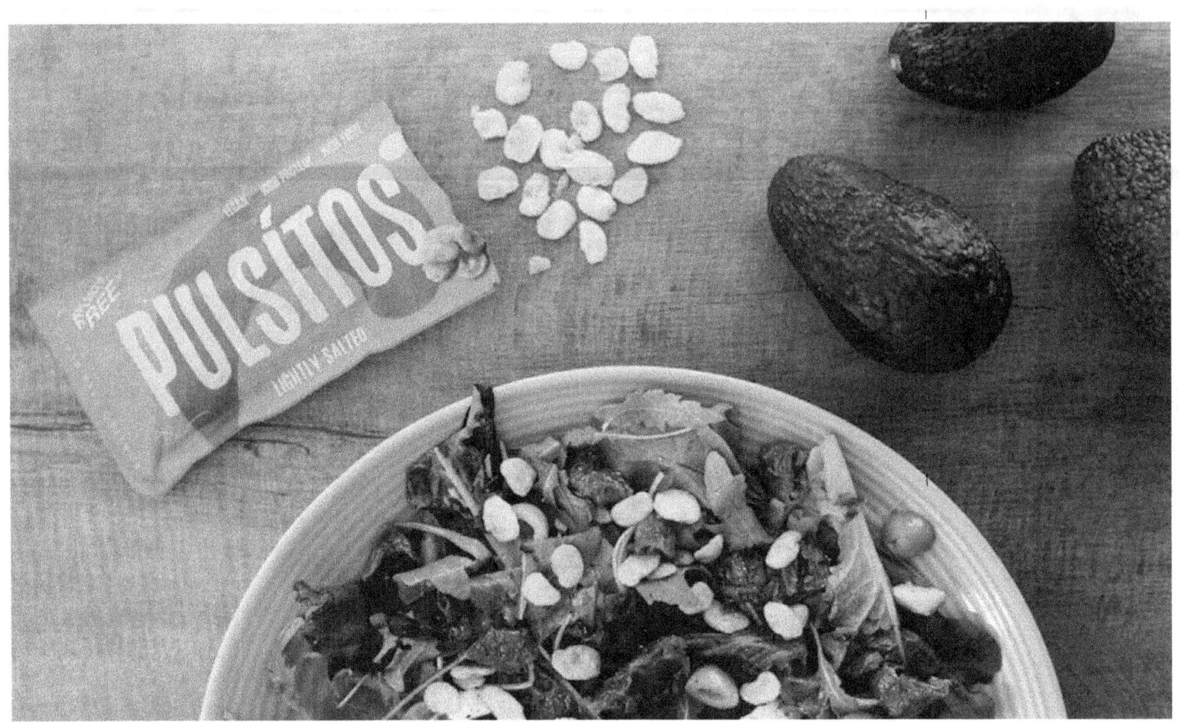

123.   Edamame Guacamole

Preparation time: 7 minutes

Cooking time: 0 minutes

Servings: 6

Ingredients:

1 cup of edamame, cooked and shelled

1 avocado, pitted and halved

½ cup of red onion, diced

¼ cup of cilantro, chopped

1 jalapeno, minced

2 cloves of garlic, minced

2 s lime juice

3 s water

½ teaspoon of lime zest

2 Roma tomato, diced

⅛ teaspoon cumin

½ teaspoon sea salt

Directions:

Into a blender or food processor add all of the ingredients, except for the diced tomato, onion, and jalapeno. Blend the tomato mixture on high speed until it is smooth and creamy, making sure that the edamame has been completely blended.

Adjust the seasoning to your preference and then transfer the guacamole to a serving bowl. Stir in the tomato, onion, and jalapeno. Place the bowl in the fridge, allowing it to chill for at least thirty minutes before serving.

Nutrition: Calories: 100, Carbs: 13g, Fat: 6g, Protein: 45g

124.   Eggplant Fries with Fresh Aioli

Preparation time: 10 minutes

Cooking time: 25 minutes

Servings: 4

Ingredients:

2 eggplants

¼ teaspoons black pepper, ground

2 s extra virgin olive oil

1 cornstarch

1 teaspoon basil, dried

¼ teaspoon garlic powder

½ teaspoon sea salt

½ cup of Mayonnaise, made with olive oil

1 teaspoon Garlic, minced

1 basil, fresh, chopped

1 teaspoon Lemon juice

½ teaspoon Chipotle, ground

¼ teaspoon sea salt

Directions:

Begin by preheating your oven to Fahrenheit four-hundred and twenty-five degrees. Place a wire cooking/cooling rack on a baking sheet.

Remove the peel from the eggplants and then slice them into rounds, each about three-quarters of an inch thick. Slice the rounds into wedges one inch in width.

Add the eggplant wedges to a large bowl and toss them with the olive oil. Once coated, add the pepper, cornstarch, dried basil, garlic powder, and sea salt, tossing until evenly coated.

Arrange the eggplant wedges on top of the wire rack and set the baking sheet in the oven, allowing the fries to cook for fifteen to twenty minutes.

Meanwhile, prepare the aioli. To do this, add the remaining ingredients into a small bowl and whisk them together to combine. Cover the bowl of aioli and allow it to chill it in the fridge until the fries are ready to be served.

Remove the fries from the oven immediately upon baking, or allow them to cook under the broiler for an additional three to four minutes for extra crispy fries. Serve immediately with the aioli.

Nutrition: Calories 243, Fat: 2g, Carbs: 12g, Protein: 5g

125.   Eggplant Caponata

Preparation time: 10 minutes

Cooking time: 25 minutes

Servings: 4

Ingredients:

1 pound of eggplant, sliced into 1.5-inch cubes

1 bell pepper, diced

½ cup of Green and black olives, chopped

¼ cup of capers

1 teaspoon of sea salt

4 garlic, minced

1 red onion, diced

15 ounces of diced tomatoes

4 s extra virgin olive oil, divided

¼ teaspoon of black pepper, ground

¼ cup of Parsley, chopped

Directions:

Preheat your oven to Fahrenheit four-hundred degrees and line a baking sheet with kitchen parchment.

Toss the eggplant cubes in half of the olive oil and then arrange them on the baking sheet, sprinkling the sea salt over the top. Allow the eggplant to roast until tender, about twenty minutes.

Meanwhile, add the remaining olive oil into a large skillet along with the red onions, bell pepper, diced tomatoes, and garlic. Sautee the vegetables until tender, about ten minutes.

Add the roasted eggplant, capers, olives, and black pepper to the skillet, continuing to cook together for five minutes so that the flavors meld.

Remove the skillet from the heat, top it off with parsley, and serve it with crusty toast.

Nutrition: Calories 129, **Fat:** 6g, **Carbs:** 12g, **Protein:** 10g

126.   Buckwheat Crackers

Preparation time: 10 minutes

Cooking time: 1 hour

Servings: 12

Ingredients:

2 cups Buckwheat groats

¾ cup Flaxseeds, ground

⅓ cup Sesame seeds

2 sweet potatoes, medium, grated

⅓ cup Extra virgin olive oil

1 cup Water

1 teaspoon Sea salt

Directions:

Soak the buckwheat groats in water for at least four hours before preparing the crackers. Once done soaking, drain off the water.

Preheat the oven to a temperature of Fahrenheit three-hundred and fifty degrees, prepare a baking sheet, and set aside some kitchen parchment and plastic wrap.

In a kitchen bowl, combine the ground flaxseeds with the warm water, allowing the seeds to absorb the water and form a substance similar to gelatin. Add the buckwheat groats and other remaining ingredients.

Spread the cracker dough onto a sheet of kitchen parchment and cover it with a sheet of plastic wrap. Use a rolling pen on top of the plastic wrap (so that it doesn't stick) and roll out the buckwheat cracker dough until it is thin.

Peel the plastic wrap off of the crackers and transfer the dough-coasted sheet of kitchen parchment to the prepared baking sheet. Allow it to partially bake for fifteen minutes and then remove the tray from the oven.

Reduce the oven temperature to Fahrenheit three-hundred degrees. Use a pizza cutter and slice the crackers into squares, approximately two inches in width. Return the crackers to the oven until they are crispy and dry, about thirty-five to forty minutes.

Remove the crackers from the oven, allowing them to cool completely before storing them in an air-tight container.

Nutrition: Calories 221, Fat: 6g, Carbs: 9g, Protein: 8g

127. Matcha Protein Bites

Preparation time: 15 minutes

Cooking time: 70 minutes

Servings: 12

Ingredients:

¼ cup Almond butter

2 teaspoons Matcha powder

1 ounce Soy protein isolate

½ cup Rolled oats

1 Chia seeds

2 teaspoons Coconut oil

1   Honey

⅛ teaspoon Sea salt

Directions:

In a food processor combine all of the matcha protein bite ingredients until it forms a mixture similar to wet sand, that will stick together when squished between your fingers.

Divide the mixture into twelve equal portions. You can do this by eye while estimating, or you can use a digital kitchen scale if you want the portions to be exact. Roll each portion between the palms of your hands to form balls.

Chill the bites in the fridge for up to two weeks.

Nutrition: Calories 165, **Fat:** 3g, **Carbs:** 6g, **Protein:** 12g

128.   Chocolate-Covered Strawberry Trail Mix

Preparation time: 5 minutes

Cooking time: 0 minutes

Servings: 10

Ingredients:

1 cup Freeze-dried strawberries

0.66 cup Dark chocolate chunks

1 cup Walnuts, roasted

¼ cup Almonds, roasted

¼ cup Cashews, roasted

Directions:

Mix together all of the trail mix ingredients in a bowl, and then store it in a large glass jar or divide each serving into its own transportable plastic bag. Store for up to one month.

Nutrition: Calories 189, Fat: 3g, Carbs: 17g, Protein: 3g

129.	Moroccan Spiced Eggs

Preparation time: 1 hour 10 minutes

Cooking time: 45 minutes

Servings: 2

Ingredients:

1 tablespoon olive oil

1 shallot, stripped and finely hacked

1 red (chime) pepper, deseeded and finely hacked

1 garlic clove, stripped and finely hacked

1 courgette (zucchini), stripped and finely hacked

1 tablespoon tomato puree (glue)

½ teaspoon gentle stew powder

¼ teaspoon ground cinnamon

¼ teaspoon ground cumin

½ teaspoon salt

400g can hacked tomatoes

400g may chickpeas in water

A little bunch of level leaf parsley cleaved

4 medium eggs at room temperature

Directions:

Heat the oil in a pan, include the shallot and red (ringer) pepper and fry delicately for 5 minutes. At that point include the garlic and courgette (zucchini) and cook for one more moment or two. Include the tomato puree (glue), flavors and salt and mix through.

Add the cleaved tomatoes and chickpeas (dousing alcohol and all) and increment the warmth to medium. With the top of the dish, stew the sauce for 30 minutes – ensure it is delicately rising all through and permit it to lessen in volume by around 33%.

Remove from the warmth and mix in the cleaved parsley.

Preheat the grill to 200C/180C fan/350F.

When you are prepared to cook the eggs, bring the tomato sauce up to a delicate stew and move to a little broiler confirmation dish.

Crack the eggs on the dish and lower them delicately into the stew. Spread with thwart and prepare in the grill for 10-15 minutes. Serve the blend in unique dishes with the eggs coasting on the top.

Nutrition: Calories 112, Fat: 5g, Carbs: 13g, Protein: 6g

130. Sirt Chili Con Carne

Preparation time: 1 hour 20 minutes

Cooking time: 1 hour 3 minutes

Servings: 4

Ingredients:

1 red onion, finely cleaved

3 garlic cloves, finely cleaved

2 10,000 foot chilies, finely hacked

1 tablespoon additional virgin olive oil

1 tablespoon ground cumin

1 tablespoon ground turmeric

400g lean minced hamburger (5 percent fat)

150ml red wine

1 red pepper, cored, seeds evacuated and cut into reduced down pieces

2 x 400g tins cleaved tomatoes

1 tablespoon tomato purée

1 tablespoon cocoa powder

300ml hamburger stock

5g coriander, cleaved

5g parsley, cleaved

160g buckwheat

Directions:

In a meal, fry the onion, garlic and bean stew in the oil over a medium heat for 2-3 minutes, at that point include the flavors and cook for a moment.

Include the minced hamburger and dark colored over a high heat. Include the red wine and permit it to rise to decrease it considerably.

You may need to add a little water to accomplish a thick, clingy consistency. Just before serving, mix in the hacked herbs.

In the interim, cook the buckwheat as indicated by the bundle guidelines and present with the stew.

Nutrition: Calories 342, Fat: 11g, Carbs: 29g, Protein: 14g

131.   Salmon and Spinach Quiche

Preparation time: 55 minutes

Cooking time: 45 minutes

Servings: 2

Ingredients:

600g frozen leaf spinach

1 clove of garlic

1 onion

150g frozen salmon fillets

200g smoked salmon

1 small Bunch of dill

1 untreated lemon

50 g butter

200 g sour cream

3 eggs

Salt, pepper, nutmeg

1 pack of puff pastry

Directions:

Let the spinach thaw and squeeze well.

Peel the garlic and onion and cut into fine cubes.

Cut the salmon fillet into cubes 1-1.5 cm thick.

Cut the smoked salmon into strips.

Wash the dill, pat dry and chop.

Wash the lemon with hot water, dry, rub the zest finely with a kitchen grater and squeeze the lemon.

Heat the butter in a pan. Sweat the garlic and onion cubes in it for approx. 2-3 minutes.

Add spinach and sweat briefly.

Add sour cream, lemon juice and zest, eggs and dill and mix well.

Season with salt, pepper and nutmeg.

Preheat the oven to 200 degrees top / bottom heat (180 degrees convection).

Grease a spring form pan and roll out the puff pastry in it and pull up on edge. Prick the dough with a fork (so that it doesn't rise too much).

Pour in the spinach and egg mixture and smooth out.

Spread salmon cubes and smoked salmon strips on top.

The quiche in the oven (grid, middle inset) about 30-40 min. Yellow gold bake.

Nutrition: Calories 320, Fat: 8g, Carbs: 18g, Protein: 12g

132. Choc Chip Granola

Preparation time: 55 minutes

Cooking time: 20 minutes

Servings: 2

Ingredients:

200g large oat flakes

Roughly 50 g pecan nuts chopped

3 tablespoons of light olive oil

20g butter

1 tablespoon of dark brown sugar

2 tablespoon rice syrup

60 g of good quality (70%)

Dark chocolate shavings

Directions:

Oven preheats to 160 ° C (140 ° C fan / Gas 3). Line a large baking tray with a sheet of silicone or parchment for baking.

In a large bowl, combine the oats and pecans. Heat the olive oil, butter, brown sugar, and rice malt syrup gently in a small non-stick pan until the butter has melted, and the sugar and syrup dissolve. Do not let boil. Pour the syrup over the oats and stir thoroughly until fully covered with the oats.

Spread the granola over the baking tray and spread right into the corners. Leave the mixture clumps with spacing, instead of even spreading. Bake for 20 minutes in the oven until golden brown is just tinged at the edges. Remove from the oven, and leave completely to cool on the tray.

When cold, split with your fingers any larger lumps on the tray and then mix them in the chocolate chips. Put the granola in an airtight tub or jar, or pour it. The granola is to last for at least 2 weeks.

Nutrition: Calories 521, **Fat:** 6g, **Carbs:** 29g, **Protein:** 18g

### 133.	Kale & Red Onion Salsa

Preparation time: 55 minutes

Cooking time: 30 minutes

Servings: 2

Ingredients:

Chicken breast

2 teaspoons ground turmeric

Lemon

Olive oil

Kale

Red onion

Ginger

Buckwheat

Directions:

Add the chili, parsley, capers, lemon juice and mix.

Preheat the oven to 220°C. Pour 1 teaspoon of the turmeric, the lemon juice and a little oil on the chicken breast and marinate. Allow to stay for 5–10 minutes.

Place an ovenproof frying pan on the heat and cook the marinated chicken for a minute on each side to achieve a pale golden color. Then transfer the pan containing the chicken to the oven and allow to stay for 8–10 minutes or until it is done. Remove from the oven and cover with foil, set aside for 5 minutes before serving.

Put the kale in a steamer and cook for 5 minutes. Pour a little oil in a frying pan and fry the red onions and the ginger to become soft but not colored. Add the cooked kale and continue to fry for another minute.

Cook the buckwheat following the packet's instructions using the remaining turmeric. Serve alongside the chicken, salsa, and vegetables.

Nutrition: Calories 129, Fat: 8g, Carbs: 19g, Protein: 9g

134.   Leek With Pine Nuts

Preparation time: 45 minutes

Cooking time: 15 minutes

Servings: 2

Ingredients:

20g Ghee

2 teaspoon Olive oil

2 pieces Leek

150 ml Vegetable broth

Fresh parsley

1 tablespoon fresh oregano

1 tablespoon Pine nuts (roasted)

Directions:

Cook the leek until golden brown for 5 minutes, stirring constantly.

Add the vegetable broth and cook for another 10 minutes until the leek is tender.

Stir in the herbs and sprinkle the pine nuts on the dish just before serving.

Nutrition: Calories 158, Fat: 6g, Carbs: 17g, Protein: 9g

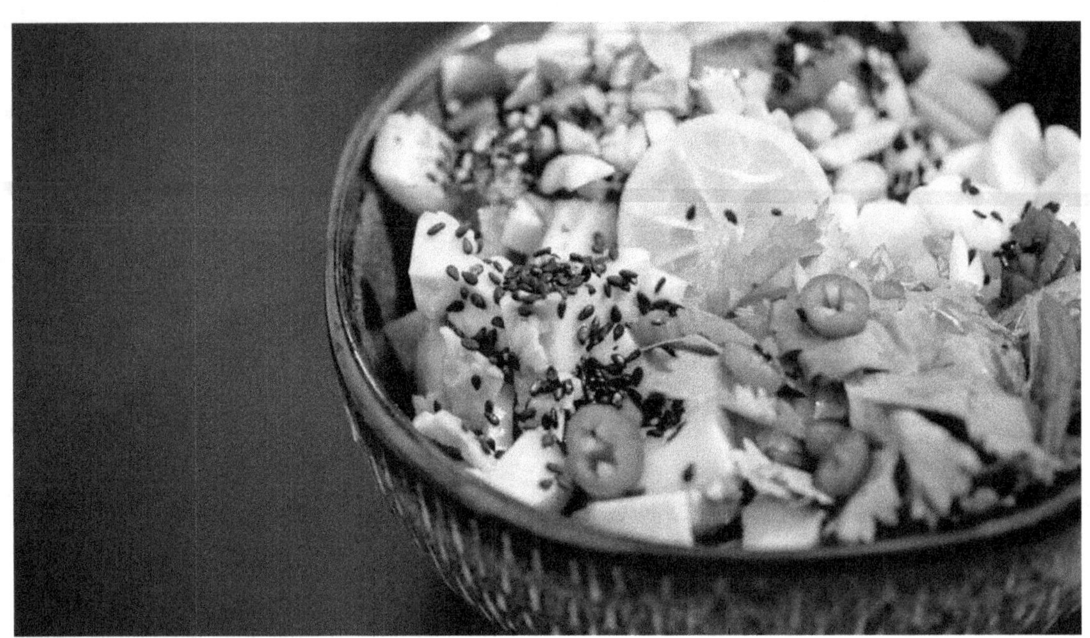

135.   Spinach Salad With Bacon

Preparation Time: 10 minutes

Cooking Time: 15 minutes

Servings: 2

Ingredients:

2 eggs

4 slices bacon

5 cups fresh spinach, rinsed and torn into bite-size pieces

½ cup sliced fresh mushrooms

1 cup sliced fresh strawberries

½ cup thinly sliced onion

1 kiwi, sliced

½ mandarin orange, peeled and segmented

1 cup seasoned croutons

Ketchup Cider Salad Dressing

Directions

Place eggs in water and bring to a boil. Take the eggs off as soon as the water boils, cover and let it sit for 12 to 15 minutes. Place in cold water. When cool, peel, chop and set the eggs aside.

Pour over the ketchup cider salad dressing and mix thoroughly.

Garnish with croutons , if desired.

Nutrition:

Calories 354, Fat: 2g, Carbs: 6g, Protein: 18g

136.   Beef And Veggies Salad

Preparation Time: 10 minutes

Cooking Time: 10 minutes

Servings: 2

Ingredients:

Boiled beet

½ onion

Cold, cooked peas

Cold, boiled carrot

Celery

Cold, boiled string beans

Cold, boiled asparagus tips

Lemon, juiced

Pourable Mayonnaise Salad Dressing (recipe in salad dressing)

Directions:

All the vegetables should be cold when making this salad. Cut the beet and half of an onion into small pieces.

Add in some asparagus tips and string beans.

Also put in some cooked peas, carrot, and celery.

Mix all this together thoroughly, and pour the mayonnaise dressing over it.

Add the juice of a lemon and serve.

Nutrition: Calories 257, Fat: 12g, Carbs: 2g, Protein: 16g

137.   Herring Cold Meat Salad

Preparation Time: 10 minutes

Cooking Time: 10 minutes

Servings: 2

Ingredients:

Salt herring

Cold slices of meat (your choice)

1 teaspoon mustard

1 beetroot

4 tablespoons oil

3 tablespoons tarragon

Vinegar

½ ounce of capers

3 boiled potatoes

Pickles (garnish)

Chopped parsley (garnish)

Small radishes (garnish)

Directions:

Wash the herring in cold water and soak it in milk for an hour.

Cut it open and clean out the bones and innards, and slice the fish and the cold meat into bite-size pieces.

Put the fish and cold meat into a salad bowl.

Chop up the capers and add them to the bowl on top of the cold meat and fish.

Mix up the mustard in a bowl or cup, gradually add the oil, and then gradually add the vinegar.

Mix this up thoroughly and then pour it over the salad and top with cold potato slices.

If you have any leftover cold vegetables, you can slice these up and garnish the salad. if not, you can use green pickles, chopped fine or a little chopped parsley, and some small radishes.

Nutrition: Calories 328, Fat: 12g, Carbs: 6g, Protein: 18g

138.	Grouse And Eggs Salad

Preparation Time: 10 minutes

Cooking Time: 10 minutes

Servings: 2

Ingredients:

8 eggs (hard-boiled)

Fresh salad greens

1 or 2 roasted grouse

Small, sweet pickles (garnish)

Anchovies (garnish)

Egg Yolk Salad Dressing (recipe in salad dressing)

Directions:

Peel the boiled eggs and cut into slices.

Cut up your cooked grouse into pieces and arrange egg slices on top.

Prepare the egg yolk salad dressing.

Lay the grouse onto the salad, and pour egg yolk salad dressing.

Lay a layer of salad, then grouse, and keep alternating until salad and grouse are gone.

In between each layer pour the sauce.

Garnish with a little bit of radish or beetroot.

Also garnish with anchovy and small pickles, cut into small pieces and placed on top of the salad.

Nutrition: Calories 411, Fat: 10g, Carbs: 2g, Protein: 21g

139.   Chicken Salad With Hard-Boiled Eggs

Preparation Time: 10 minutes

Cooking Time: 10 minutes

Servings: 2

Ingredients:

Chicken

Cucumber

2 heads of lettuce

2 boiled beets

Boiled eggs

Cayenne Mustard Salad Dressing (recipe in salad dressings)

Directions:

Shred the chicken in a bowl.

Chop up the cucumber and beet and put it with the chicken.

Toss lightly.

Pour the chicken salad dressing over the salad.

Toss lightly again to coat evenly.

Garnish with slices of hard-boiled eggs.

Nutrition: Calories 280, Fat: 2g, Carbs: 1g, Protein: 16g

140.   Chicken With Nut And Fruit Salad

Preparation Time: 10 minutes

Cooking Time: 10 minutes

Servings: 2

Ingredients:

2 large fresh peaches

2 cups chopped, cooked chicken meat

½ cup thinly sliced red onion

½ cup Poppy Seed Mayo Salad

6 cups mixed salad greens

½ cup toasted walnuts, chopped

Directions:

Put onion and chicken in a bowl.

Add in 1 peach chopped into ½ inch pieces.

Add in the onion and the salad greens with the peaches and chicken.

Add the poppy seed salad dressing and toss to coat evenly.

Transfer everything to a large serving platter or individual salad bowls.

Garnish with peach slices.

Nutrition: Calories 265, Fat: 9g, Carbs: 1g, Protein: 12g

141.   Southern Western Chicken Salad

Preparation Time: 10 minutes

Cooking Time: 0 minutes

Servings: 2

Ingredients:

2 (6 inch) flour tortillas, cut into ½-inch strips

Butter-flavored nonstick cooking spray

1 teaspoon olive oil

6 cups ready-to-serve salad greens

1 can whole kernel corn, drained

1 can black beans, rinsed and drained

Tomatoes

⅔ cup ranch salad dressing

4 teaspoons barbecue sauce

Directions:

Spritz the tortilla strips with butter flavored cooking spray, both sides. Bake at 350 degrees F for 4-5 minutes, until crispy.

Meanwhile, cook chicken over medium heat until juices are clear and it is no longer pink inside. Set aside to let cool.

Take the chicken and place it in the center of the vegetables and greens.

Garnish with remaining cheese and tomatoes.

Place the tortilla chips around the chicken.

Mix together the barbecue sauce and ranch dressing.

Put in a bowl and serve with the salad.

Nutrition: Calories 189, Fat: 2g, Carbs: 4g, Protein: 22g

142.   Chicken And Cucumber Salad

Preparation Time: 10 minutes

Cooking Time: 0 minutes

Servings: 2

Ingredients:

The remains of cold roast chicken or boiled chicken

2 heads of lettuce

A tiny bit of endive

1 cucumber

A few slices of boiled beetroot

Cayenne Mustard Salad Dressing (recipe in salad dressing)

Directions:

Cut up the chicken, diced, cubed or strips.

Wash and dry the lettuce, tear into bite size pieces, and place on a dish.

Put the pieces of chicken on top, and pour the salad-dressing over them.

Serve immediately.

Nutrition: Calories 278, Fat: 2g, Carbs: 6g, Protein: 6g

143.   Kale, Apple, & Cranberry Salad

Preparation Time: 15 minutes

Cooking Time: 15 minutes

Servings: 4

Ingredients:

6 cups fresh baby kale

3 large apples, cored and sliced

¼ cup unsweetened dried cranberries

¼ cup almonds, sliced

2 tablespoons extra-virgin olive oil

1 tablespoon raw honey

Salt and ground black pepper, to taste

Directions:

In a salad bowl, place all the ingredients and toss to coat well.

Serve immediately.

Nutrition: Calories 344, Fat: 6g, Carbs: 5g, Protein: 9g

144.   Chicken And Celery Salad

Preparation Time: 10 minutes

Cooking Time: 1 hour 30 minutes

Servings: 2

Ingredients:

2 cups chicken

1 cup diced celery

1 green pepper

French dressing

Lettuce

Easy Mayo Salad Dressing (recipe in salad dressing)

1 pimiento

Directions:

Pick the chicken off the bone and dice it.

Dice up the celery.

Take out the seeds from the green pepper, wash, and cut into small pieces.

Put the celery and pepper in with the chicken.

Marinate with French dressing, chill, and wait for about ½ hour.

Drain the marinade from the salad mixture. Serve on salad bowls garnish with a bed of lettuce leaves.

Pour salad dressing and mix thoroughly.

Garnish with strips of the pimiento.

Nutrition: Calories 305, Fat: 10g, Carbs: 2g, Protein: 8g

145.	Chicken Beet Salad

Preparation Time: 10 minutes

Cooking Time: 0 minutes

Servings: 2

Ingredients:

Chicken

1 cucumber

2 heads of lettuce

2 beets (boiled)

Dress with Cayenne Mustard Salad Dressing (recipe in salad dressing)

Directions:

Mix above ingredients, except beets, and coat with your salad dressing.

Place in salad bowls and garnish with beets.

Nutrition: Calories 180, Fat: 12g, Carbs: 3g, Protein: 20g

146.	Chicken Beetroot Salad

Preparation Time: 10 minutes

Cooking Time: 0 minutes

Servings: 2

Ingredients:

Leftover cold roast or boiled chicken

2 heads of lettuce

1 cucumber

A few slices of boiled beetroot

Salad-dressing (your choice)

Directions:

Cut up the chicken and lettuce and place on a salad platter.

Pour the salad-dressing over lettuce and chicken.

Tosss to coat evenly.

This salad should be served immediately.

Nutrition: Calories 290, Fat: 10g, Carbs: 2g, Protein: 18g

147.   Strawberry, Apple & Arugula Salad

Preparation Time: 15 minutes

Cooking Time: 0 minutes

Servings: 4

Ingredients:

4 cups fresh baby arugula

2 apples, cored and sliced

1 cup fresh strawberries, hulled and sliced

¼ cup walnuts, chopped

4 tablespoons olive oil

Salt and ground black pepper, as required

Directions:

For the salad: place all the ingredients in a large bowl and mix well.

For the dressing: place all the ingredients in a bowl and beat until well combined.

Pour the dressing over the salad and toss it all to coat well.

Serve immediately.

Nutrition: Calories 243, Fat: 19g, Carbs: 12g, Protein: 6g

148.Raspberry & Kale Salad

Preparation Time: 15 minutes

Cooking Time: 0 minutes

Servings: 2

Ingredients:

For Salad:

3 cups fresh baby kale

½ cup fresh raspberries

¼ cup walnuts, chopped

For Dressing:

1 tablespoon extra-virgin olive oil

1 tablespoon apple cider vinegar

½ teaspoon pure maple syrup

Salt and ground black pepper, as required

Directions:

For salad: in a salad bowl, place all ingredients and mix.

For dressing: place all ingredients in another bowl and beat until well combined.

Place dressing on top of the salad and toss to coat well.

Serve immediately.

Nutrition: Calories 226, Fat: 16g, Carbs: 4g, Protein: 8g

149. Mixed Berries Salad

Preparation Time: 15 minutes

Cooking Time: 0 minutes

Servings: 4

Ingredients:

Strawberries

Blackberries

Blueberries

Raspberries

6 cups fresh arugula

2 tablespoons extra-virgin olive oil

Salt and ground black pepper, as required

Directions:

In a salad bowl, place all the ingredients and toss to coat well.

Serve immediately.

Nutrition: Calories 108, Fat: 7g, Carbs: 10g, Protein: 2g

Preparation Time: 15 minutes

Cooking Time: 0 minutes

Servings: 4

Ingredients:

3 large oranges, peeled

2 beets, trimmed, peeled and sliced

6 cups fresh rocket

¼ cup walnuts, chopped

3 tablespoons olive oil

Pinch of salt

Directions:

In a salad bowl, place all ingredients and gently, toss to coat.

Serve immediately.

Nutrition: Calories 233, Fat: 15g, Carbs: 23g, Protein: 4g

Preparation Time: 15 minutes

Cooking Time: 0 minutes

Servings: 2

Ingredients:

For Salad:

3 cups fresh kale, tough ribs removed and torn

1 orange, peeled and segmented

1 grapefruit, peeled and segmented

2 tablespoons unsweetened dried cranberries

For Dressing:

2 tablespoons extra-virgin olive oil

2 tablespoons fresh orange juice

1 teaspoon Dijon mustard

½ teaspoon raw honey

Salt and ground black pepper, as required

Directions:

For salad: in a salad bowl, place all ingredients and mix.

For dressing: place all ingredients in another bowl and beat until well combined.

Place dressing on top of the salad and toss to coat well.

Serve immediately.

Nutrition: Calories 239, Fat: 13g, Carbs: 22g, Protein: 4g

152. Cucumber & Onion Salad

Preparation Time: 10 minutes

Cooking Time: 0 minutes

Servings: 4

Ingredients:

3 large cucumbers, sliced thinly

½ cup red onion, sliced

2 tablespoons olive oil

1 tablespoon fresh apple cider vinegar

Sea salt, to taste

¼ cup fresh parsley, chopped

Directions:

In a salad bowl, place all the ingredients and toss to coat well.

Serve immediately.

Nutrition: Calories 122, Fat: 5g, Carbs: 7g, Protein: 3g

153.Strawberry, Orange & Arugula Salad

Preparation Time: 15 minutes

Cooking Time: 0 minutes

Servings: 4

Ingredients:

For Salad:

6 cups fresh baby arugula

1½ cups fresh strawberries, hulled and sliced

2 oranges, peeled and segmented

For Dressing:

2 tablespoons fresh lemon juice

1 tablespoon raw honey

2 teaspoons extra-virgin olive oil

1 teaspoon Dijon mustard

Salt and ground black pepper, as required

Directions:

For salad: in a salad bowl, place all ingredients and mix.

For dressing: place all ingredients in another bowl and beat until well combined.

Place dressing on top of salad and toss to coat well.

Serve immediately.

Nutrition: Calories 234 Fat: 4g, Carbs: 9g, Protein: 4g

154.Chicken & Kale Salad

Preparation Time: 20 minutes

Cooking Time: 18 minutes

Servings: 4

Ingredients:

For Chicken:

1 teaspoon dried thyme

½ teaspoon garlic powder

½ teaspoon onion powder

¼ teaspoon cayenne pepper

¼ teaspoon ground turmeric

Salt and ground black pepper, as required

2 (7-ounce) boneless, skinless chicken breasts, pounded into ¾-inch thickness

1 tablespoon olive oil

For Salad:

6 cups fresh kale, tough ribs removed and chopped

2 cups carrots, peeled and cut into matchsticks

¼ cup walnuts

<u>For Dressing:</u>

1 small garlic clove, minced

2 tablespoons fresh lime juice

2 tablespoons extra-virgin olive oil

1 teaspoon raw honey

½ teaspoon Dijon mustard

Salt and ground black pepper, as required

Directions:

Preheat your oven to 425 °F.

Line a baking dish with parchment paper.

For chicken: in a bowl, mix together the thyme, spices, salt and black pepper.

Drizzle the chicken breasts with oil and then rub with spice mixture generously.

Arrange the chicken breasts onto the prepared baking dish.

Bake for approximately 16 - 18 minutes.

Remove the baking dish from oven and transfer chicken breasts onto a cutting board for about 5 minutes.

For salad: place all ingredients in a salad bowl and mix.

For dressing: place all ingredients in another bowl and beat until well combined.

Cut each chicken breast into desired sized slices.

Place the salad onto each serving plate and top each with chicken slices.

Drizzle with dressing and serve.

Nutrition: Calories 330, Fat: 18g, Carbs: 16g, Protein: 25g

155.Chicken & Berries Salad

Preparation Time: 20 minutes

Cooking Time: 16 minutes

Servings: 8

Ingredients:

2 pounds boneless, skinless chicken breasts

½ cup olive oil

¼ cup fresh lemon juice

2 tablespoons maple syrup

1 garlic clove, minced

Salt and ground black pepper, as required

2 cups fresh strawberries, hulled and sliced

2 cups fresh blueberries

10 cups fresh baby arugula

Directions:

In a large resealable plastic bag, place the chicken and ¾ cup of marinade.

Seal bag and shake to coat well.

Refrigerate overnight.

Cover the bowl of remaining marinade and refrigerate before serving.

Preheat the grill to medium heat. Grease the grill grate.

Remove the chicken from bag and discard the marinade.

Place the chicken onto grill grate and grill, covered for about 5 - 8 minutes per side.

Remove chicken from grill and cut into bite-sized pieces.

In a large bowl, add the chicken pieces, strawberries and spinach and mix.

Place the reserved marinade and toss to coat.

Serve immediately.

Nutrition: Calories 355, Fat: 6g, Carbs: 29g, Protein: 9g

156.   Beef & Kale Salad

Preparation Time: 15 minutes

Cooking Time: 8 minutes

Servings: 2

Ingredients:

For Steak:

2 teaspoons olive oil

2 (4-ounce) strip steaks

Salt and ground black pepper, as required

For Salad:

¼ cup carrot, peeled and shredded

¼ cup cucumber, peeled, seeded and sliced

¼ cup radish, sliced

¼ cup cherry tomatoes halved

3 cups fresh kale, tough ribs removed and chopped

<u>For Dressing:</u>

1 tablespoon extra-virgin olive oil

1 tablespoon fresh lemon juice

Salt and ground black pepper, as required

Directions:

For steak: in a large heavy-bottomed wok, heat the oil over high heat and cook the steaks with salt and black pepper for about 3 - 4 minutes per side.

Transfer the steaks onto a cutting board for about 5 minutes before slicing.

For salad: place all ingredients in a salad bowl and mix.

For dressing: place all ingredients in another bowl and beat until well combined.

Cut the steaks into desired sized slices against the grain.

Place the salad onto each serving plate.

Top each plate with steak slices.

Drizzle with dressing and serve.

157. Chicken Salad

Preparation time: 5 Minutes

Cooking Time: 30 Minutes

Servings: 2

Ingredients:

½ red onion, very finely sliced

1 tablespoon of sesame seeds

150g of cooked chicken-shredded

Large handful 20g of parsley-chopped

100g of baby kale-chopped roughly

2 teaspoons of soy sauce

1 teaspoon of clear honey

1 teaspoon of sesame oil

Directions:

Place a frying pan over medium heat and toast the sesame seeds in the dry pan for 2 minutes until they are light brown and fragrant. Transfer them to a plate and allow them to cool.

Mix the sesame oil, honey, olive oil, lime juice, and soy sauce to make the dressing.

Place the cucumber, red onion, kale, pak choi, and parsley in a large bowl and gently mix. Pour the dressing over and mix again.

Split the salad into two plates and place the shredded chicken on top.

Just before serving, sprinkle the sesame seeds.

158. Chicken with Mole Salad

Preparation time: 5 Minutes

Cooking Time: 40 Minutes

Servings: 2

Ingredients:

1 skinned chicken breast

2 cups spinach, washed, dried and torn in halves

2 celery stalks, chopped or sliced thinly

½ cup arugula

½ small red onion, diced

2 Medjool pitted dates, chopped

1 tablespoon of. of dark chocolate powder

1 tablespoon of. extra virgin olive oil

2 tablespoon of. water

5 sprigs of parsley, chopped

Dash of salt

Directions:

In a food processor, blend the dates, chocolate powder, oil and water, and salt. Add the chili and process further. Rub this paste onto the chicken breast, and set it aside, in the refrigerator.

Prepare other salad mixings, the vegetables and herbs in a bowl and toss.

Cook the chicken in a dash of oil in a pan, until done, about 10 - 15 minutes over a medium burner.

When done, let cool and lay over the salad bed and serve.

Nutrition: Calories 323, **Fat:** 6g, **Carbs:** 9g, **Protein:** 9g

159. Smoked Salmon Sirt Salad

Preparation time: 10 Minutes

Cooking Time: 40 Minutes

Servings: 4

Ingredients:

1 cup, or ¼ package if large of smoked salmon slices no cooking needed!

1 avocado, pitted, sliced, and scooped out

10 walnuts, chopped

5 lovage or celery leaves), chopped

2 celery stalks, chopped or sliced thinly

½ small red onion, sliced thinly

1 Medjool pitted date, chopped

1 tablespoon of. capers

1 tablespoon of. extra virgin olive oil

¼ of a lemon, juiced

5 sprigs of parsley, chopped

Directions:

Wash and dry salad makings and vegetables, top with salmon.

Nutrition: Calories 559, Fat: 6g, **Carbs:** 29g, **Protein:** 9g

160. Carrot, Buckwheat, Tomato & Arugula Salad in a Jar

Preparation time: 5 Minutes

Cooking Time: 30 Minutes

Servings: 2

Ingredients:

½ cup sunflower seeds

½ cup carrots½ cup of shredded cabbage

½ cup of tomatoes

1 cup cooked buckwheat mixed with 1 tablespoon of. chia seeds1 cup arugula

Dressing1 tablespoon of. olive oil 1 tablespoon of. fresh lemon juice and a pinch of sea salt

Directions:

Put ingredients in this order: dressing, sunflower seeds, carrots, cabbage, tomatoes, buckwheat and arugula.

Nutrition: Calories 165, Fat: 2g, Carbs: 6g, Protein: 4g

161. Chickpeas, Onion, Tomato & Parsley Salad in a Jar

Preparation time: 5 Minutes

Cooking Time: 50 Minutes

Servings: 2

Ingredients:

1 cup cooked chickpeas

½ cup chopped tomatoes½ of a small onion, chopped

1 tablespoon of. chia seeds1 Tablespoon of. chopped parsley

Dressing1 tablespoon of. olive oil and 1 tablespoon of. of Chlorella.1 tablespoon of. fresh lemon juice and a pinch of sea salt

Directions:

Put ingredients in this order: dressing, tomatoes, chickpeas, onions and parsley.

Nutrition: Calories 234, Fat: 15g, Carbs: 20g, Protein: 6g

162. Kale & Feta Salad with Cranberry Dressing

Preparation time: 5 Minutes

Cooking Time: 30 Minutes

Servings: 2

Ingredients:

250g 9oz kale, finely chopped

50g 2oz walnuts, chopped

75g 3oz feta cheese, crumbled

1 apple, peeled, cored and sliced

4 medjool dates, chopped

For the Dressing

75g 3ozcranberries

½ red onion, chopped

3 tablespoons olive oil

3 tablespoons water

2 teaspoons honey

1 tablespoon red wine vinegar

Sea salt

Directions:

Place the ingredients for the dressing into a food processor and process until smooth. If it seems too thick, you can add a little extra water if it is necessary. Place all the ingredients for the salad into a bowl.

Pour on the dressing and toss the salad until it is well coated in the mixture.

Nutrition: Calories 342, Fat: 6g, Carbs: 18g, Protein: 9g

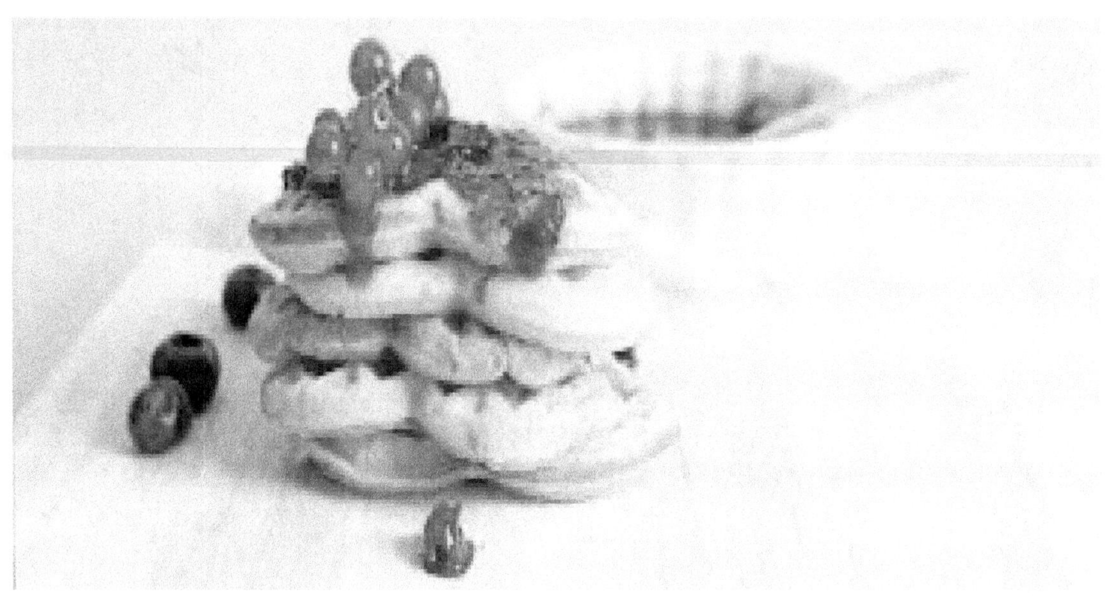

163.   Sirtfood Truffle Bites

Preparation time: 1 hour

Cooking time: 0 min

Servings: 15-20 pcs

Ingredients:

1 cup walnuts

¾ cup of Medjool dates, pitted

½ cup of dark chocolate broken into pieces; or cocoa nibs

2 heaping tablespoons of cacao powder

½ cup of dried coconut

1 tablespoon of. ground turmeric

1 tablespoon of. extra virgin olive oil or coconut oil (preferred)

1 teaspoon of. vanilla extract, or a vanilla pod, scraped

1 dash of cayenne pepper

1 dash sea salt (up to ⅛ teaspoon)

2 tablespoon of. water if needed

Directions:

Pulse in a food processor the walnuts and chocolate until finely pulverized. Gently blend solid ingredients next and the vanilla. Make a dough. Make rolled balls out of the dough. Add water a few drops at a time only if it is necessary.

Do not use too much water, or you will have to go and add more of the other ingredients to compensate. Refrigerate. Store for up to a week.

Take them with you to work or when traveling for a quick pick-me-up as well as to quell a sweet tooth.

Nutrition: Calories 256, Fat: 12g, Carbs: 6g, Protein: 9g

164.   Spicy Kale Chips

Preparation time: 2 hours 15 minutes

Cooking time: 15 minutes

Servings: 1

Ingredients:

1 large head of curly kale, wash, dry, and pulled from stem 1 tablespoon of. extra virgin olive oil

Minced parsley

Lemon juice

Cayenne pepper (just a pinch)

Dash of soy sauce

Directions:

In a large bowl, rip the kale from the stem into palm-sized pieces. Sprinkle the minced parsley, olive oil, soy sauce, a squeeze of the lemon juice, and a very small pinch of the cayenne powder. Toss with a set of tongs or salad forks, and make sure to coat all of the leaves.

If you have a dehydrator, turn it on to 118 F, spread out the kale on a dehydrator sheet, and leave it there for about 2 hours.

If you are cooking them, place parchment paper on top of a cookie sheet, lay the bed of kale, and separate it a bit to make sure the kale is evenly toasted. Cook for 10-15 minutes maximum at 250F.

Nutrition: Calories 321, **Fat:** 10g, **Carbs:** 2g, **Protein:** 9g

165.   Sweet and Savory Guacamole

Preparation time: 20 minutes

Cooking time: 0 minutes

Servings: 2

Ingredients:

2 large avocados, pitted and scooped

2 Medjool dates, pitted and chopped into small pieces

½ cup cherry tomatoes cut into halves

5 sprigs of parsley, chopped

¼ cup of arugula, chopped

5 sticks of celery, washed, cut into sticks for dipping

Juice from ¼ lime

Dash of sea salt

Directions:

Mash the avocado in a bowl, sprinkle salt, and squeeze of the lime juice. Fold in the tomatoes, dates, herbs, and greens. Scoop with celery sticks, and enjoy!

Nutrition: Calories 218, Fat: 6g, Carbs: 9g, Protein: 9g

166.   Thai Nut Mix

Preparation time: 30 minutes

Cooking time: 20 minutes

Servings: 1

Ingredients:

½ cup walnuts

½ cup coconut flakes

½ teaspoon of. soy sauce

1 teaspoon of. honey

1 pinch of cayenne pepper

1 dash of lime juice

Directions:

Add the above ingredients to a bowl, toss the nuts to coat, and place on a baking sheet, lined with parchment paper. Cook at 250 F for 15-20 minutes, checking as not to burn, but lightly toasted.

Remove from the oven. Cool first before eating.

Nutrition: Calories 322, Fat: 6g, Carbs: 2g, Protein: 6g

167.   Berry Yogurt Freeze

Preparation time: 1 hour 30 minutes

Cooking time: 0 minutes

Servings: 2

Ingredients:

2   cups plain yogurt (Greek, soy or coconut)

½ cup sliced strawberries

½ cup blackberries

1 teaspoon of. honey (warmed) ½ teaspoon of. chocolate powder

Directions:

Blend all of the above ingredients until creamy in a bowl. Place into two glass or in metal bowls that are freezer-safe, and put into the freezer for 1 hour, remove and thaw just slightly so that it is soft enough to eat with a spoon, makes two servings.

Nutrition: Calories 229, Fat: 6g, Carbs: 2g, Protein: 5g

168.   Summer Berry Smoothie

Preparation time: 20 minutes

Cooking time: 0 minutes

Servings: 1

Ingredients:

Blueberries

Strawberries

Blackcurrants

Red grapes

1 carrot, peeled

1 orange, peeled

Juice of 1 lime

Directions:

Place all of the ingredients into a blender and cover them with water. Blitz until smooth. You can also add some crushed ice and a mint leaf to garnish.

Nutrition: Calories 232, Fat: 5g, Carbs: 2g, Protein: 9g

169.   Buckwheat Pancakes with Strawberries and Chocolate Nut Butter

Preparation time: 25 minutes

Cooking Time: 25 minutes

Servings: 8

Ingredients:

1.5 cups soy milk

1 cup buckwheat flour

1 large egg

1 tablespoon extra-virgin olive oil, for cooking

1 ½ cups strawberries, chopped

For the chocolate nut butter:

⅔ cup dark chocolate (at least 85%)

¼ cup milk

2 tablespoons double cream

1 tablespoon coconut oil

½ cup walnuts

Directions:

Place milk, flour, and egg in a blender and blend until smooth. Transfer batter to measuring cup for easy pouring. To make the chocolate nut butter: melt chocolate in a double-boiler, once melted, whisk in the milk, then the double cream and oil. Pour into a blender with your walnuts and blend until smooth. For a saucier mix, add more milk or cream as desired.

To make the pancakes: warm a griddle to medium heat, adding a small amount of oil as needed. Pour batter onto griddle and cook until lightly browned on the bottom.

Watch for air bubbles. You will know it's time to flip your pancake when the air bubbles pop. Flip your pancakes and cook until lightly browned on the other side. Repeat with the remaining batter. Top pancakes with strawberries and drizzle over with sauce, as desired.

Nutrition: Calories 321, Fat: 4g, Carbs: 2g, Protein: 8g

170.   Blackcurrant and Raspberry Jelly

Preparation Time: 8 minutes

Cooking Time: 7 minutes

Servings: 2

Ingredients:

½ cup Raspberries, washed

½ cup Blackcurrants, washed and stalks removed

2 Leaves of Gelatin

300ml of Water

2 Tablespoon Granulated Sugar

Directions:

Share the raspberries into two serving glasses or dishes. Soften the gelatin leaves by placing them in a bowl of cold water.

Place the blackcurrants in a small pan; add 100ml of water and the sugar. Allow to boil, and then simmer vigorously for five minutes before you put off the heat. Allow standing for two minutes.

Squeeze out any excess water from the leaves, and then add them to the saucepan. Stir together until fully dissolved, then add the rest of the water and stir. Pour the liquid into the serving glasses or dishes and place in the refrigerator to set, best to refrigerate overnight or a minimum of 3 to 4 hours.

Nutrition: Calories 348, Fat: 4g, Carbs: 2g, Protein: 3g

171.   Apple Pancakes with Blackcurrant Compote

Preparation Time: 20 minutes

Cooking Time: 20 minutes

Servings: 4

Ingredients:

2 Egg whites

1 cup Plain flour

½ cup Porridge oats

1 teaspoon Baking powder

Pinch of salt

2 tablespoon Caster sugar

2 Apples, peeled, cored and chopped into small pieces

2 teaspoon Light olive oil

300ml Semi-skimmed milk

For the Compote:

½ cup Blackcurrant, washed and stalks removed

3 tablespoons Water

2 tablespoons Caster sugar

Directions:

The first step is to get your compote ready. Add the water, sugar, and blackcurrant into a small pan. Allow to simmer, and then cook for about 10 to 15 minutes. Add the baking powder, salt, caster sugar, flour, and oats in a large bowl. Mix thoroughly. Add the apples, stir, and then whisk in the milk, a little at a time until you have a smooth consistency.

Whisk the egg whites to stiff peaks then add into the pancake batter. Move the batter into a jug. Heat half teaspoon of oil in a non-stick frying pan over medium-high heat. Begin by pouring in approximately one-quarter of the batter. Cook on both sides until the batter turns golden brown. Remove the set and add the next batch until you have four pancakes. Place the pancakes in a plate and drizzle the blackcurrant compote over them. Serve.

Nutrition: Calories 332, Fat: 5g, Carbs: 2g, Protein: 8g

172. Chocolate Chip Cookies

Preparation Time: 7 minutes

Cooking Time: 10 minutes

Servings: 10

Ingredients*:*

½ cup Semi-sweet chocolate chips

½ teaspoon Baking soda

½ teaspoon Vanilla

1 Egg

1 cup Flour

½ cup Margarine

4 teaspoons Stevia

Directions:

Sift the dry ingredients.

Cream the margarine, stevia, vanilla and egg with a whisk.

Add flour mixture and beat well.

Stir in the chocolate chips, then drop teaspoonful of the mixture over a greased baking sheet.

Bake the cookies for about 10 minutes at 375F.

Cool and serve.

Nutrition: Calories 108, Fat**:** 7g, Carbs**:** 8g, Protein**:** 9g

173.	Herbed Mixed Nuts

Preparation Time: 10 minutes

Cooking Time: 25 minutes

Servings: 12

Ingredients:

1 tablespoon of. butter, melted

1 tablespoon of. Worcestershire sauce

2 teaspoon ofs. dried basil and/or oregano, crushed

½ teaspoon of. garlic salt

3 cups walnuts, soy nuts, and/or almonds

2 tablespoon ofs. grated Parmesan cheese

Directions:

Set an oven to preheat to 325 degrees F.

Mix together the garlic salt, herb, Worcestershire sauce and melted butter in a bowl, then add nuts and mix until coated.

Use foil to line a 15x10x1-inch baking pan, then spread the nuts in the pan. Put parmesan on top, then stir until coated.

Let it bake for 15 minutes, mixing two times. Allow it to cool. Tightly cover and store up to a maximum of one week.

Nutrition: Calories 222, Fat: 2g, Carbs: 16g, Protein: 2g

174.   Cinnamon Graham Popcorn

Preparation Time: 10 minutes

Cooking Time: 30 minutes

Servings: 3

Ingredients:

2-½ quarts popped popcorn

2 cups Golden Grahams

1-½ cups golden raisins

1 cup chopped dates

1 cup miniature marshmallows

⅓ cup butter, melted

¼ cup packed brown sugar

2 teaspoon ofs. ground cinnamon

½ teaspoon of. ground ginger

½ teaspoon of. ground nutmeg

Directions:

Mix marshmallows, dates, raisins, cereal, and popcorn together in a big bowl.

Mix the rest of the ingredients together. Put on the popcorn mixture and mix to blend.

Put in two oiled 15x0x1-in. baking pans.

Bake without a cover at 250°, tossing 1 time, about 20 minutes. Preserve in an airtight container.

Nutrition: Calories 243, Fat: 1g, Carbs: 12g, Protein: 3g

175.   Cucumber Bites

Preparation Time: 10 minutes

Cooking Time: 0 minutes

Servings: 12

Ingredients:

1 English cucumber, sliced into 32 rounds

10 ounces hummus

16 cherry tomatoes, halved

1 tablespoon parsley, chopped

1 ounce feta cheese, crumbled

Directions:

Spread the hummus on each cucumber round, divide the tomato halves on each, sprinkle the cheese and parsley on to and serve as an appetizer.

Nutrition: Calories 119, Fat: 1g, Carbs: 3g, Protein: 18g

Preparation Time: 10 minutes

Cooking Time: 15 minutes

Servings: 16

Ingredients:

1½ teaspoon ofs. brown sugar

¼ to ½ teaspoon of. salt

¼ teaspoon of. ground red pepper

Directions:

Set an oven to preheat to 350 degrees F. Spread the almonds or pecans on the baking tray in a single layer.

Let it bake for around 10 minutes or until it becomes aromatic and a bit toasted.

In the meantime, melt the margarine or butter in a medium saucepan on medium heat until it sizzles. Take it out of the heat. Stir in red pepper, salt, sugar and rosemary.

Add the nuts to the butter mixture and toss until coated.

Allow it to cool a bit prior to serving.

Nutrition: Calories 190, Fat: 1g, Carbs: 18g, Protein: 2g

177.   Plum & Pistachio Snack

Preparation Time: 5 minutes

Cooking Time: 5 minutes

Servings: 1

Ingredients:

¼ cup unsalted dry-roasted pistachios (measured in shell)

1 plum

Directions:

Hull and serve pistachios together with plum.

Nutrition: Calories 113, Fat: 2g, Carbs: 6g, Protein: 9g

178.	Wrapped Plums

Preparation Time: 5 minutes

Cooking Time: 0 minutes

Servings: 8

Ingredients:

Prosciutto

4 plums, quartered

1 tablespoon chives, chopped

Red pepper flakes

Directions:

Wrap each plum quarter in a prosciutto slice, arrange them all on a platter and serve.

Nutrition: Calories 260, Fat: 1g, Carbs: 8g, Protein: 4g

179.	Chocolate Coconut Macaroons

Preparation Time: 10 minutes

Cooking Time: 40 minutes

Servings: 20

Ingredients:

2 eggs

½ cup sugar

Salt

1 oz. dark chocolate, chopped and melted

Directions:

Set oven to 350°F to preheat. Line parchment paper over a large rimmed baking sheet.

In a medium bowl, beat egg whites until they form soft peaks using an electric mixer. Add sugar and keep beating until egg whites become glossy. Mix in salt, vanilla (or almond) extract, and coconut. Shape the mixture into balls, about 1 tablespoon of. each, making 20 balls in total; transfer the balls to the prepared baking sheet.

Bake macaroni for 15 to 20 minutes in the preheated oven until the inside is soft and the outside is browned lightly. Allow to cool on a wire rack.

Ladle melted chocolate into a small plastic bag. Cut off a very small tip of one corner. Pipe melted chocolate through the slit and drizzle over the cooled cookies. Another way, plunge a fork into melted chocolate and instantly a draw a wave over the cookies.

Allow the cookies to sit until chocolate is set before preserving or serving them.

Nutrition: Calories 244, Fat: 2g, Carbs: 8g, Protein: 4g

180.   Lemonade Stand

Preparation Time: 5 minutes

Cooking Time: minutes

Servings: 9

Ingredients:

3 cups animal crackers

2 cups salted peanuts

2 cups raisins

2 cups milk chocolate

Directions:

Mix all ingredients in a big bowl, then store in snack-size resealable plastic bags.

Nutrition: Calories 213, Fat: 1g, Carbs: 10g, Protein: 4g

181. Sideline Snackers

Preparation Time: 15 minutes

Cooking Time: 15 minutes

Servings: 3

Ingredients:

3 quarts popped popcorn

2 cups pretzel sticks

2 cups salted peanuts

1-¼ teaspoon ofs. chili powder

¾ teaspoon of. paprika

½ teaspoon of. garlic salt

¼ teaspoon of. onion salt

¼ teaspoon of. ground mustard

¼ teaspoon of. ground cumin

6 tablespoon ofs. butter, melted

Directions:

Mix peanuts, pretzels and popcorn in a big bowl. Mix seasonings.

Sprinkle butter atop popcorn mixture and put seasonings on top; toss to cover.

Keep in sealed container.

Nutrition: Calories 190, Fat: 2g, Carbs: 1g, Protein: 10g

Preparation Time: 15 minutes

Cooking Time: 10 minutes

Servings: 8

Ingredients:

6 cups water

2 ¼ teaspoon ofs. salt

2 cups yellow grits

1 stick of butter

½ teaspoon of. black pepper

2 tablespoon ofs. garlic

½ lb Cheddar

3 eggs

1 cup milk

Directions:

In center position, put oven rack; preheat the oven to 350°F.

Boil ¾ teaspoon of. salt and water in 4-qt. heavy pot.

In a slow stream, add grits, constantly mixing; lower heat. Gently simmer, frequently mixing to avoid sticking, for 30 minutes till very thick. To avoid popping hot grits and bubbling, use long-handled spoon.

Add cheese, garlic, pepper, leftover 1 ½ teaspoon of. salt and butter, mixing till cheese and butter melt.

Put into ungreased 8-in. 2-in. deep square baking dish; bake for 1 hour till lightly browned and set. Immediately serve.

Nutrition: Calories 320, Fat: 1g, Carbs: 2g, Protein: 4g

183.   Blueberry Pancakes

Preparation Time: 5 minutes

Cooking Time: 10 Minutes

Servings: 2

Ingredients*:*

½ teaspoon baking powder

1 egg white

¼ cup soy milk

¼ tablespoon honey

⅛ cup blueberries

1 tablespoon olive oil

Directions:

Sift together flour and baking powder, set aside.

Beat together the egg white, milk, and honey in a bowl.

Stir in flour until just moistened, add blueberries, and stir to incorporate.

Preheat a heavy-bottomed skillet over medium heat, and spray with cooking spray. 5. Pour approximately ¼ teaspoon of the olive oil into the pan for each pancake.

Cook until bubbly, turn and continue cooking until golden brown.

Nutrition: Calories 122, Fat: 6g, Carbs: 7g, Protein: 8g

Preparation Time: 10 Minutes

Cooking Time: 25 Minutes

Servings: 4

Ingredients:

¾ cup stevia

2 cups coconut milk

3 tablespoons flaxseed mixed with 4 tablespoons water

Juice of 2 limes

Zest of 1 lime, grated

1 cup cherries, pitted and halved

1 cup cauliflower rice

Directions:

In a pan, combine the milk with the stevia and bring to a simmer over medium heat.

Add the cauliflower rice and the other ingredients, stir, cook for 25 minutes more, divide into cups and serve cold.

Nutrition: Calories 199, Fat: 5g, Carbs: 11g, Protein: 5g

185.	Ginger Avocado Kale Salad

Preparation Time: 15 Minutes

Cooking Time: 0

Servings: 4

Ingredients:

1 avocado, peeled and sliced

1 tablespoon of. ginger, grated

½ lb. kale, chopped

¼ cup parsley, chopped

2 fresh scallions, chopped

Directions:

Add all ingredients into the mixing bowl and toss well.

Serve and enjoy.

Nutrition: Calories 233, Fat: 5g, Carbs: 6g, Protein: 8g

186.   Refreshing Cucumber Salad

Preparation Time: 10 Minutes

Cooking Time: 0

Servings: 4

Ingredients:

⅓ cup cucumber basil ranch

1 cucumber, chopped

3 tomatoes, chopped

3 tablespoon of. fresh herbs, chopped

½ onion, sliced

Directions:

Add all ingredients into the large mixing bowl and toss well.

Serve immediately and enjoy.

Nutrition: Calories 184, Fat: 3g, Carbs: 12g, Protein: 3g

Preparation Time: 15 Minutes

Cooking Time: 0

Servings: 4

Ingredients:

⅓ cup unsweetened desiccated coconut

½ medium head cabbage, shredded

2 teaspoon of. sesame seeds

¼ cup tamari sauce

¼ cup olive oil

1 fresh lemon juice

½ teaspoon of. cumin

½ teaspoon of. curry powder

½ teaspoon of. ginger powder

Directions:

Add all ingredients into the large mixing bowl and toss well.

Place salad bowl in refrigerator for 1 hour.

Serve and enjoy.

Nutrition: Calories 197, Fat: 2g, Carbs: 4g, Protein: 5g

Preparation Time: 20 Minutes

Cooking Time: 0

Servings: 4

Ingredients:

2 avocados, diced

4 cups cabbage, shredded

3 tablespoon of. fresh parsley, chopped

2 tablespoon of. apple cider vinegar

4 tablespoon of. olive oil

1 cup cherry tomatoes, halved

½ teaspoon of. pepper

1 ½ teaspoon of. sea salt

Directions:

Add cabbage, avocados, and tomatoes to a medium bowl and mix well.

In a small bowl, whisk together oil, parsley, vinegar, pepper, and salt.

Pour dressing over vegetables and mix well.

Serve and enjoy.

Nutrition: Calories 253, Fat: 21g, Carbs: 14g, Protein: 3g

189.   Turnip Salad

Preparation Time: 10 Minutes

Cooking Time: 0

Servings: 4

Ingredients:

4 white turnips, spiralized

1 lemon juice

4 dill sprigs, chopped

2 tablespoon of. olive oil

1 ½ teaspoon of. salt

Directions:

Season spiralized turnip with salt and gently massage with hands.

Add lemon juice and dill. Season with pepper and salt.

Drizzle with olive oil and combine everything well.

Serve immediately and enjoy.

Nutrition: Calories 49, Fat: 1g, Carbs: 9g, Protein: 1g

190.   Sassy Chocolate Mousse

Preparation Time: 10 Minutes

Cooking Time: 0

Servings: 4

Ingredients:

Coconut cream scraped from the upper side of 2 pieces of 13.5-ounce chilled cans of full fat coconut milk

4 tablespoons of cocoa

3 tablespoons of Agave Nectar

1 teaspoon of vanilla extract

Directions:

Take a large bowl and scoop out the thick coconut cream from the can to the bowl

Add nectar, vanilla extract and cocoa to the bowl

Beat it well using an electric mixer, starting from low and going to medium until a foamy texture appears

Divide the mix evenly amongst ramekins and chill to your desired level of cold

Enjoy!

Nutrition: Calories 134, Fat: 3g, Carbs: 14g, Protein: 4g

191.   Tender Heirloom Carrots

Preparation Time: 10 Minutes

Cooking Time: 45 Minute

Servings: 3-4

Ingredients:

1 bunch heirloom carrots

1 tablespoon of fresh thyme leaves

½ a tablespoon of coconut oil

1 tablespoon of maple syrup

⅛ cup of fresh squeeze orange juices

⅛ teaspoon of sea salt

Salt as needed

Directions:

Pre-heat your oven to 350-degree Fahrenheit

Wash your carrots well and discard any green pieces

Take a small sized mixing bowl and add coconut oil, maple syrup, orange juice and a bit of salt

Pour the mixture over your carrots and spread on a large sized baking sheet

Sprinkle a bit of thyme and roast for 45 minutes

Sprinkle a generous amount of salt and a bit of thyme as garnish

Enjoy!

Nutrition: Calories 70, Fat: 3g, Carbs: 4g, Protein: 3g

192.   Raspberry Brule

Preparation Time: 15 minutes

Cooking Time: 1 minute

Servings: 4

Ingredients:

½ cup Light sour cream

½ cup Plain cream cheese

¼ cup Brown sugar, divided

¼ teaspoon of Ground cinnamon

1 cup Fresh raspberries

Directions:

Preheat the oven to broil.

In a bowl, beat together the cream cheese, sour cream, 2 tablespoon of. brown sugar and cinnamon for 4 minutes or until the mixture is very smooth and fluffy.

Evenly divide the raspberries among 4 (4-ounce) ramekins.

Spoon the cream cheese mixture over the berries and smooth the tops.

Sprinkle ½ tablespoon of. brown sugar evenly over each ramekin.

Place the ramekins on a baking sheet and broil 4 inches from the heating element until the sugar is caramelized and golden brown.

Cool and serve.

Nutrition: Calories 188, Fat: 6g, Carbs: 2g, Protein: 9g

193.   Baked Carrot Pudding

Preparation Time: 15 minutes

Cooking Time: 30 Minutes

Servings: 4

Ingredients*:*

1 egg white

½ tablespoon honey

⅛ teaspoon vanilla extract

¼ teaspoon baking powder

⅛ cup all-purpose flour

Directions:

Blend the soy milk and chia seeds together in a blender.

Pour mixture into 4 clear dessert dishes. Stir to evenly distribute the chia seeds.

Refrigerate until set, about 1 hour in the refrigerator or ½ hour in the freezer.

Top each serving with 1 tablespoon of shredded coconut, 1 large strawberry and 1 tablespoon of blueberries before serving.

Nutrition: Calories 559, Fat: 6g, Carbs: 29g, Protein: 9g

194.   Dessert Crepes

Preparation Time: 10 minutes

Cooking Time: 10 Minutes

Servings: 4

Ingredients*:*

1 egg white, lightly beaten

¼ cup soy milk

½ tablespoon butter, melted

½ cup all-purpose flour

¼ tablespoon honey

Directions:

Cook over medium heat, 1 to 2 minutes on a side, or until golden brown. Serve immediately.

Nutrition: Calories 213, Fat: 6g, Carbs: 2g, Protein: 6g

195.   Fig Duff

Preparation Time: 20 minutes

Cooking Time: 180 Minutes

Servings: 6

Ingredients:

½ cup graham crackers crumbs

¼ teaspoon baking powder

⅛ teaspoon ground cinnamon

¼ teaspoon ground nutmeg

⅛ teaspoon ground cloves

½ tablespoon butter

⅛ cup soy milk

1 egg white, beaten

¼ cup honey

Directions:

In a large bowl, stir together the graham crackers crumbs, baking powder, cinnamon, nutmeg and cloves.

Preheat the oven to 250 degrees F. Grease a large pudding mold. Place the mold into another larger baking dish, place the pudding mold and dish into the oven, then fill the outer dish with at least 1 inch of water.

Steam for 4 hours in the preheated oven, or until the pudding is firm. Cool slightly before removing from the mold. Best served with a lemon hard sauce.

Nutrition: Calories 231, Fat: 4g, Carbs: 2g, Protein: 5g

196.   Lemon Chiffon Pudding

Preparation Time*:* 15 minutes

Cooking Time*:* 35 Minutes

Servings: 6

Ingredients*:*

3 ½ tablespoons all-purpose flour

⅔ cup honey

2 tablespoons butter, softened

3 tablespoons lemon juice

⅔ cup soy milk

2 egg whites

Directions:

Preheat the oven to 350 degrees F (175 degrees C).

In a large bowl, stir together the flour and honey until well blended. Stir in butter until smooth. Gradually beat in lemon juice and soy milk. Fold egg whites into the lemon mixture. Transfer to a casserole dish.

Bake for 35 minutes in the preheated oven, or until set. Serve warm or chilled.

Nutrition: Calories 213, Fat: 6g, Carbs: 3g, Protein: 8g

197.	Grapefruit Squares

Preparation Time*:* 15 minutes

Cooking Time*:* 10 Minutes

Servings: 6

Ingredients*:*

1 cup honey (divided use)

1 cup all-purpose flour

½ cup unsalted butter

½ teaspoon baking powder

2 egg whites, slightly beaten

4 tablespoons grapefruit juice (divided use)

1 tablespoon unsalted butter, softened

1 tablespoon lemon peel

Directions:

To make crust mix together ¼ cup honey, flour and ½ cup butter.

Pour into ungreased 8" square pan and bake at 350 degrees F for 15 minutes. Remove from oven.

To make filling mix together honey, baking powder, beaten egg whites, 2 tablespoons grapefruit juice and grated lemon peel.

Pour over crust and spread evenly.

Return to oven and bake 20 minutes longer at 350 degrees F. Remove from oven and cool.

To make icing mix together remaining 2 tablespoons grapefruit juice, ¾ cup honey and 1 tablespoon softened butter.

When crust and filling layers are completely cool.

Nutrition: Calories 159, **Fat:** 6g, **Carbs:** 8g, **Protein:** 9g

198.   Cheese Cookies

Preparation Time: 15 minutes

Cooking Time: 10 Minutes

Servings: 6

Ingredients:

2 cups honey

1 cup unsalted butter

15 ounces cream cheese

2 teaspoon vanilla extract

2 large egg whites

1 tablespoon lemon juice

4 cups all-purpose flour

1-½ teaspoons baking soda

3 tablespoons soy milk

Directions

Preheat the oven to 350 degrees F. Set butter out to soften.

In a large bowl using a hand-mixer on low speed, beat together honey and butter. Blend well. Increase the speed to high; beat until light and fluffy, about 5 minutes.

With the mixer on medium speed mix in the cream cheese, vanilla, egg whites and lemon juice. Set mixer to low speed and add flour, baking soda. Beat until a dough form.

Drop by tablespoons onto an ungreased cookie sheet, spaced about 2-inches apart. Bake for 15 minutes, or until slightly golden brown.

Remove from the oven and cool cookies completely on a wire rack.

Nutrition: Calories 459, Fat**:** 6g, Carbs**:** 4g, Protein**:** 9g

199.   Jam Cake

Preparation Time: 25 minutes

Cooking Time*:* 60 Minutes

Servings: 6

Ingredients:

1 cup butter

1 cup honey

2 egg whites

1 teaspoon baking soda

3 cups all-purpose flour

1 cup soymilk

1 cup blackberry

Directions:

Preheat oven to 350 degrees F. Lightly grease one 10-inch tube pan and set aside.

Cream together the butter and honey. Add egg whites separately, beating well after each.

Sift together soda and flour; add alternately with milk to creamed mixture. Mix well. Serve

Nutrition: Calories 421, Fat: 6g, Carbs: 2g, Protein: 2g

200.   Lemon Mousse

Preparation Time: 10 + chill time

Cooking Time: 10 minutes

Servings: 4

Ingredients*:*

1 cup coconut cream

8 ounces cream cheese, soft

¼ cup fresh lemon juice

3 pinches salt

1 teaspoon lemon liquid stevia

Directions:

Preheat your oven to 350 °F

Grease a ramekin with butter

Beat cream, cream cheese, fresh lemon juice, salt and lemon liquid stevia in a mixer

Pour batter into ramekin

Bake for 10 minutes, then transfer the mousse to a serving glass

Let it chill for 2 hours and serve

Enjoy!

Nutrition: Calories 332, Fat: 6g, Carbs: 1g, Protein: 9g

201. Fruit Trifle

Preparation Time*:* 35 minutes

Cooking Time*:* 5 Minutes

Servings: 4

Ingredients*:*

8 oz. biscuits, chopped

¼ cup strawberries, chopped

1 banana, chopped

1 peach, chopped

½ mango, chopped

1 cup grapes, chopped

1 tablespoon liquid honey

1 cup of orange juice

½ cup Plain yogurt

¼ cup cream cheese

1 teaspoon coconut flakes

Directions:

Bring the orange juice to boil and remove it from the heat.

Add liquid honey and stir until it is dissolved.

Cool the liquid to the room temperature.

Add chopped banana, peach, mango, grapes, and strawberries. Shake the fruits gently and leave to soak the orange juice for 15 minutes.

Meanwhile, with the help of the hand mixer mix up together Plain yogurt and cream cheese.

Then separate the chopped biscuits, yogurt mixture, and fruits on 4 parts.

Place the first part of biscuits in the big serving glass in one layer.

Spread it with yogurt mixture and add fruits. Repeat the same steps till you use all ingredients.

Top the trifle with coconut flakes.

Nutrition: Calories 390, Fat: 8g, Carbs: 2g, Protein: 6g

Over the course of this book, you have not only learned the basic information required to start the Sirtfood diet; you have gained much more than that! By learning how to meal plan, prep, and storage, you will be able to easily master the Sirt food diet with little day-to-day effort required. You will be able to enjoy delicious meals at a moment's notice without having to struggle after a long day of work. By just preparing a little ahead of time, you can have a fridge and freezer fully stocked with delicious homemade meals perfectly suited to your taste.

The Sirtfood Diet is based on research on sirtuins, a group of proteins that regulate several functions in the body. Certain foods called sirtfoods may cause the body to produce more of these proteins. This diet may help you lose weight because it's low in calories, but the weight is likely to return once the diet ends. The Sirtfood Diet consists of two phases. Phase 1 lasts seven days and combines calorie restriction and green juices, while Phase 2 lasts two weeks and includes three meals and one juice.

Sirtfood diet works through a unique concept that has proven to be effective through repeated experiments. We have many practical examples which indicate that sirtfood can actually help you lose weight and boost your metabolism. If you were new to this idea, then this cookbook must have provided you have the relevant and much-needed information in a concise and precise manner. It's about time to give all its Sirtfood recipes a try and see the results after progressively controlling your diet over the two phases.

Sirtfoods are typically healthy foods. However, very little is known about how these foods affect sirtuin levels and human health. The Sirtfood Diet promotes healthy foods but is restrictive in calories and food choices. It also involves drinking lots of juice, which isn't a healthy recommendation. The Sirtfood Diet is low in calories, and phase one is not nutritionally balanced. It may leave you hungryy, but the Sirtfood Diet is full of healthy foods thus it's not dangerous for the average healthy adult.

Furthermore, the majority of the top sirtfoods are fruits, vegetables, and plant-based foods. When combined with the right amount of proteins and carbohydrates in your daily meals, then you cannot go wrong by eating more of them than you usually do. Just remember to keep your red wine, caffeine, and dark chocolate in moderation to avoid causing unintentional harm to your body.

Finally, as a rule of thumb, you should not put your 100% trust on a diet that has promises that sound a bit too good to be true. Set realistic expectations based on your current situation in life. Not everyone can live like Adele and the other celebrity endorsers of the Sirtfood Diet.

The menu plan I provided you will help you get on your feet. Whether you choose to use the plan exactly how I designed, customize it, or create your own from scratch, you will find that by having a plan and guide to follow eating healthier, losing weight and boosting your health can be easier than ever.